THE HEALTH PROFESSIONAL'S

HPV HANDBOOK

1: HUMAN PAPILLOMAVIRUS AND CERVICAL CANCER

Editors-in-Chief
Professor Walter Prendiville
Coombe Women's Hospital, Dublin, Ireland

Dr Philip Davies
European Consortium for Cervical Cancer Education,
London, UK

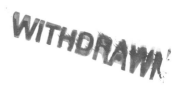

THE HEALTH PROFESSIONAL'S

HPV HANDBOOK

1: HUMAN PAPILLOMAVIRUS AND CERVICAL CANCER

Editors-in-Chief

Professor Walter Prendiville
Coombe Women's Hospital, Dublin, Ireland

Dr Philip Davies
European Consortium for Cervical Cancer Education,
London, UK

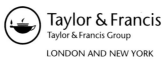

Taylor & Francis
Taylor & Francis Group

LONDON AND NEW YORK

A PARTHENON BOOK

First published in the United Kingdom in 2004
by Taylor & Francis,
an imprint of the Taylor & Francis Group,
2 Park Square, Milton Park
Abingdon, Oxon OX14 4RN, UK

Tel.:   +44 (0) 20 7017 6000
Fax.:   +44 (0) 20 7017 6699
Website: www.tandf.co.uk

ISBN 1-84214-336-0

Composition by Parthenon Publishing
Printed and bound by T.G. Hostench, S.A., Spain

The European Consortium for Cervical Cancer Education is supported by a grant from the
European Commission: No. QLG4-CT-2001-30142, and in part by unconditional
educational grants from Roche Molecular Systems and Digene Europe.

The publishing and printing costs of these handbooks were defrayed by an unrestricted
educational grant from Roche Molecular Systems.

No commercial organization had any involvement in the writing, editing or approval of
these books.

Contents

List of contributors

F Xavier Bosch
Institut Catala d'Oncologia,
L'Hospitalet de Llobregat,
Epidemiology and Cancer
Registration, Barcelona, Spain

Xavier Castellsagué
Institut Catala d'Oncologia,
L'Hospitalet de Llobregat,
Epidemiology and Cancer
Registration, Barcelona, Spain

Philip Davies
European Consortium for
Cervical Cancer Education,
London, UK

Thomas Hiller
Sektion Experimentelle Virologie,
Universitätsklinikum Tübingen,
Elfriede-Aulhorn Strasse,
Tübingen, Germany

Thomas Iftner
Sektion Experimentelle Virologie,
Universitätsklinikum Tübingen,
Elfriede-Aulhorn Strasse,
Tübingen, Germany

Fiona Lyons
Department of Genitourinary
Medicine and Infectious
Diseases, St James's Hospital,
Dublin, Ireland

Niamh Murphy
Department of Pathology,
Coombe Women's Hospital and
Trinity College, Dublin, Ireland

John O'Leary
Department of Pathology,
Coombe Women's Hospital,
Department of Histopathology,
St James's Hospital and
Trinity College, Dublin, Ireland

Toli S Onon
Department of Immunology,
Paterson Institute for Cancer
Research, Christie Hospital,
Manchester, UK

Walter Prendiville
Coombe Women's Hospital,
Dublin, Ireland

Martina Ring
Department of Pathology,
Coombe Women's Hospital and
Trinity College, Dublin, Ireland

Sílvia de Sanjosé
Institut Catala d'Oncologia,
L'Hospitalet de Llobregat,
Epidemiology and Cancer
Registration, Barcelona, Spain

Orla Sheils
Department of Histopathology,
St James's Hospital and
Trinity College, Dublin, Ireland

Introduction to the HPV Handbook series

These compact, illustrated handbooks are concise but comprehensive resources that introduce medical students, general medical practitioners and gynaecologists to the significance of the human papillomaviruses in the etiology of cervical cancer. All chapters are fully referenced and written by experts in the field.

Handbook 1: *Human Papillomavirus and Cervical Cancer*, introduces the human papillomaviruses that are responsible for genital warts or cervical cancer. The chapters review virus structure, the epidemiology of HPV, the latest advances in HPV vaccination and new markers for cervical disease.

Handbook 2: *Current Evidence-based Applications*, describes the implications of implementing HPV testing for the management of women with various degrees of dysplasia, and discusses HPV testing for post-treatment follow-up. It also provides an overview of the current status of HPV testing as a tool for cervical cancer screening.

Handbook 3: *HPV and Cervical Cancer: Public Health Perspectives*, examines the benefits and drawbacks of cervical cytology and HPV testing as part of an organized screening programme to prevent cervical cancer.

1. The human papillomavirus

Thomas Hiller and Thomas Iftner

- Human papillomaviruses (HPVs) can cause benign or malignant disease

- The majority of infections are without symptoms

- The viral origin of cervical cancer is proven beyond any reasonable doubt

- High-risk (HR) and low-risk (LR) genotypes can be distinguished by DNA sequence differences in certain genes

- Progress has been made in defining the molecular basis of oncogenesis

Introduction

Human papillomaviruses (HPVs) belong to the family Papovaviridae. They consist of a 72-capsomere capsid containing the viral genome.[1] The capsomeres are made of two structural proteins: the 57 kD late protein L1, which accounts for 80% of the viral particle, and the 43–53 kD minor capsid protein L2. HPVs are relatively stable and, because they have no envelope, remain infectious in a moist environment for months.[2]

Papillomaviruses are widespread among higher vertebrates but exhibit a strict species specificity, and transmission from non-primates to humans has not been reported. In general, they cause local epithelial infections, with the exception of animal fibropapilloma viruses, where the infection can also be found in the dermis. A viremia with viral spread to distant body sites does not occur.

Classification of papillomaviruses

Human papillomaviruses were originally classified into cutaneous types such as HPV 1, 4, 10, etc. and mucosal types such as HPV 6, 16, 31, etc. However, this classification proved too simple and was incorrect in some cases, as demonstrated by the presence of the mucosal type HPV 6 in cornifying genital warts. Another attempt to group papillomaviruses was the separation into skin types causing vulgar warts – for example, HPV 1 and the genital types primarily affecting the anogential area (e.g. HPV 6, 16, 18). Again, this classification was artificial because HPV 16 can also be found in nail-bed carcinoma of the hands.

Clinical presentation

Infections with HPVs may cause local cell proliferation, which can develop into plantar or common warts and condylomas. The majority of these benign tumours regress spontaneously in immunocompetent individuals. However, in those with inherited or pharmacologically

Modern HPV classification

- Based on DNA sequence differences within the coding regions of the early proteins E6, E7 and the late protein L1

- Genotypes have < 90% DNA sequence homology in these regions; over 130 have been described, to date
  - Subtypes have 90–98% homology within a genotype
    - Variants have ≥ 98% homology within a subtype

induced immune deficiencies, there is a strong tendency for the infections to persist, with a high probability of malignancy in the case of infection with high-risk (HR) HPV types.

The malignant potential of HPV-induced papillomas was first demonstrated in patients with the rare hereditary disease, Epidermodysplasia verruciformis (EV). In these patients, several EV-specific HPV types induce disseminated warts. Within 20 years of disease onset, 30–60% of EV patients are predicted to develop squamous cell carcinoma, primarily at sun-exposed sites. More than 90% of these carcinomas contain HPV 5 DNA, and the majority of the remainder HPV 8 DNA.

The viral origin of cervical cancer has now been proven beyond any reasonable doubt.[3–5] Recent studies have shown that HPV DNA can be found in 99.7% of all cervical carcinomas, with HPV types 16, 18, 45 and 31 being the most frequent.[6,7] Based on these observations, the anogenital HPVs have been divided into two groups: the first is associated with a high risk for cervical cancer development – the HR HPVs (16, 18, 26, 31, 33, 35, 39, 45, 51, 52, 53, 56, 58, 59, 66, 68, 73 and 82), and the second group with a low carcinogenic potential – the low-risk (LR) HPVs (6, 11, 40, 42, 43, 44, 54, 61, 72 and 81).[8] It has now been proven beyond reasonable doubt that infection with an HR HPV is a necessary prerequisite for the development of cervical cancer, and the World Health Organization (WHO) has recognized HPV 16 and HPV 18 as carcinogenic agents for humans.

Clinical associations of HPV genotypes

- Warts of the skin (HPV 1–4, 7, 10, 26–29, 41, 48, 49, 57, 60, 63, 65)
  - Verruca plantaris/plantar warts, mosaic-type warts, verruca plana/flat warts, butchers' warts
- Upper respiratory tract and eye (HPV 2, 6, 11, 13, 16, 32)
  - Laryngeal papilloma, recurrent respiratory, papillomatosis, nasal papilloma, oral papilloma, focal epithelial hyperplasia, conjunctival papilloma
- Epidermodysplasia verruciformis (HPV 5, 8–9, 12, 14, 15, 17, 19, 20–25, 36, 38, 47, 50)
  - Macular lesions
  - Squamous cell carcinoma
- Anogenital warts (HPV 2, 6, 11, 16, 18, 30, 40–42, 44, 45, 54, 55, 61)
  - Condylomata accuminata, flat condylomata, Bowen's disease, Buschke-Loewenstein tumours
- Anogenital carcinomas – the HR HPVs (HPV 16, 18, 26, 31, 33, 35, 39, 45, 51, 52, 53, 56, 58, 59, 66, 68, 73, 82)
  - Squamous cell carcinoma of the cervix, vulva and penis
  - Squamous cell carcinoma of the remaining anogenital tract

Structure of the HPV genome

The HPV genome consists of eight kilobasepairs (Kbp), and is a double-stranded DNA molecule. The relative arrangement of the 8–10 open reading frames (ORFs) within the genome is the same in all papillomavirus types, and a particular characteristic of papilloma-viruses is that the partly overlapping ORFs are arranged on only one DNA strand. The genome can be divided into three regions: the long control region (LCR) without coding potential; the region of early proteins (E1–E8); and the region of late proteins (L1 and L2).

An example of the genome organization of human papillomaviruses is shown in Figure 1.

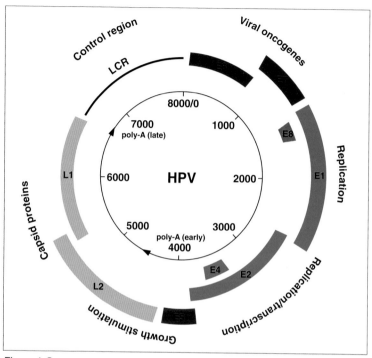

Figure 1 Genome organization of human papillomaviruses

The proteins of papillomaviruses

The sizes and functions of papillomavirus proteins are shown in Table 1. E6 and E7 are the most important oncogenic proteins. Transcription of the E6 and E7 genes was observed always to occur in cervical carcinomas, and this was the first indication of an important role for these genes in HPV-associated tumourigenesis.[9,10] The immortalizing and transforming potential of E6 and E7 proteins have been demonstrated in numerous experiments, both in tissue culture as well as experimental animal models.[11,12]

E8^E2 fusion protein

Recently, a new E2 protein, consisting of a fusion of the product of the small E8 ORF with part of the E2 protein, has been described. This fusion protein is able to repress viral DNA replication as well as transcription, and is therefore believed to play a major role in the maintenance of viral latency observed in the basal cells of infected epithelium.[13,14]

Table 1 Size and function of papillomavirus proteins

Viral protein/ genomic element	Molecular weight/size	Function
Non-coding elements		
Long control region (LCR)	500-1000 bp	Origin of replication and regulation of HPV gene expression
Early proteins		
E1	68–85 kD	Helicase function; essential for viral replication and control of gene transcription; similar among types
E2	48 kD	Viral transcription factor; essential for viral replication and control of gene transcription; genome segregation and encapsidation
E3	Unknown	Function not known; only present in a few HPVs
E1^E4	10–44 kD	Binding to cytoskeletal protein
E5	14 kD	Interaction with EGF/PDGF-receptors
E6	16–18 kD	Interaction with several cellular proteins; degradation of p53 and activation of telomerase
E7	~ 10 kD	Interaction with several cellular proteins; interaction with pRB and transactivation of E2F-dependent promoters
E8^–E2C	20 kD	Long distance transcription and replication repressor protein
Late proteins		
L1	57 kD	Major capsid protein
L2	43–53 kD	Minor capsid protein

The E6 protein: Key action is p53 inhibition

The E6 ORF encodes a small protein of approximately 150 amino acids with a molecular weight of 16–18 kD. The E6 protein of HR anogenital types shows only weak oncogenic potential in most established cell lines and cooperation with the E7 protein is required for full transforming and immortalizing capacity.

The key action of HR E6 proteins is the inhibition of the function of p53, a tumour suppressor protein, by enhancing its degradation through the ubiquitin pathway.[15–19] To inhibit p53, E6 requires a cellular protein called E6-associated protein (E6AP). In non-infected cells, the ubiquitin-mediated degradation of p53 is triggered by the mdm-2 protein, while in HR HPV-infected cells the E6-E6AP complex replaces mdm-2 in the control of cellular p53 levels (Figure 2).[15] This shift dramatically shortens the p53 half-life from 3 hours to 20 minutes, decreases biological function, and reduces p53 protein level in cervical carcinoma cells to less than half the level found in normal epithelial cells.[20] Most E6 proteins from LR HPVs do not bind to p53, and none of them induce its degradation.

HR HPV E6 proteins lead to a down-regulation of p53-dependent transcription, independently of E6AP-dependent degradation of the p53 protein. Furthermore, the E6 protein appears to activate the cellular enzyme telomerase in differentiated cells. Telomerase counteracts the continuous shortening of the chromosome telomeres during replication of the cellular genome. This shortening is correlated with cell ageing, and the prevention of chromosome shortening results in an increased life-span of the affected cell.

The E7 protein: The major transforming protein of HPV

The E7 ORF encodes for a small protein of approximately 100 amino acids with a molecular weight of 10 kD. E7 is the major transforming oncogene of HPVs and it acts by binding cellular proteins of the pRB tumour suppressor family, which, by interacting with the E2F-family of transcription factors, control cell replication.[21] Binding of E7 to the active form of pRB leads to the release of E2F transcription factors,

SPRING CREEK CAMPUS

which then stimulate entry into the S-phase of the cell cycle and lead to cell replication (Figure 2).[22] This interaction induces multiple cellular responses, including attempts to stabilize the p53 protein that would normally counter the stimulated cell replication by increasing apoptosis (programmed cell death).[23] However, as noted above, the HR HPV E6 protein increases the degradation of p53 and thereby blocks the cellular response.

It is currently unclear how LR papillomaviruses (whose E6 proteins are unable to interfere with p53 but whose E7 proteins bind to pRB) overcome the p53-mediated apoptosis. In addition, it has been shown that the E6 proteins of some HPV types bind to a component of the single-strand break DNA repair complex and thereby inhibit its efficiency.[24] A cell that is persistently infected with HPV, therefore, undergoes continuous cell division, and consequently is no longer able to react in response to DNA damage with G1 arrest or apoptosis.

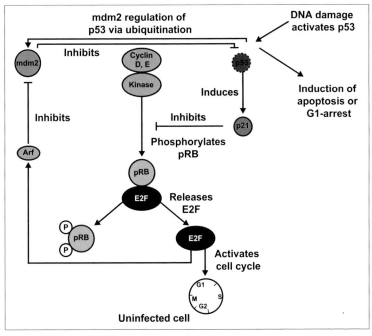

Figure 2 Effect of E6/E7 on cell proliferation

DNA repair is also impeded, which clearly promotes the cell's pathway to malignancy.

LR anogenital HPV types, such as HPV 6, are unable to degrade p53. Therefore, the capability of anogenital E6 and E7 proteins to degrade p53 or pRb would seem to correlate with their oncogenic potential. Such a correlation has not been demonstrated for the cutaneous papillomaviruses; the E6 proteins of HPV 5 and HPV 8, for example, are unable to bind or degrade p53. Since cutaneous and LR genital HPVs have E7 proteins that bind to pRB but do not affect p53 by E6-mediated degradation, they seem to follow another pathway to overcome E7-induced cell defence mechanisms. Consequently, the search for further cellular partners of E6 and E7 proteins is ongoing. Tables 2 and 3 summarize the known interactions of E6 and E7 proteins and the possible consequences of these interactions for infected cells.

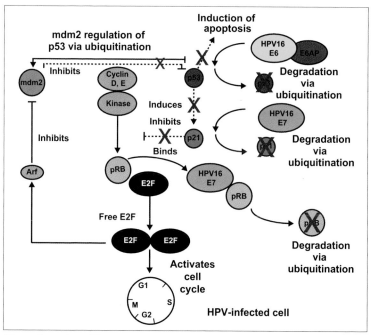

Figure 2 *continued* Effect of E6/E7 on cell proliferation

Table 2 Cellular binding partners for E6

Cellular binding partner	Cellular function of the binding partner	Degradation (+/–)	Possible consequences of interaction for the cell
AMF-1/ Gps2	Enhances p300 activity	+	Suppression of Gps2; transcriptional activation activity
Bak	Member of Bcl-2 family; pro-apoptotic protein	+	Anti-apoptotic effect
CBP/ p300	p53 co-activator; regulation of signal-modulating events (activation of genes for cell-cycle control, differentiation, immune response)	–	Down-regulation of p53-dependent transcription
c-myc	Transcription factor; induction of apoptosis	+	To counter myc-induced apoptosis?
E6AP	Regulation of signal transduction in proliferating cells via degradation of the src family kinase Blk	+	Deregulation of signal transduction in proliferating cells; essential factor for degradation actions of the E6-protein
E6TPI	GAP-protein (GTPase-activating protein) – negative regulator of Rab	+	Inhibition of Rab-mediated mitogenic signalling
ERC55 (E6BP)	Calcium-binding protein (has a role in epithelial cell differentiation and inhibition of apoptosis)	–	Inhibition of terminal differentiation of epithelial cells; p53-independent inhibition of apoptosis
hDLG/ Sap97	Human homologue to the drosophila discs large tumour suppressor protein important in formation of polarities in epithelial cell differentiation, formation and maintenance of tight junctions	+	Affects cell adhesion, polarity and proliferation, contributing to the invasiveness of the transformed cell?
hScrib	Expressed in epithelial tight junctions; human homologue to the drosophila tumour suppressor protein Scrib (which controls formation of cell junctions and inhibition of epithelial cell growth)	+	Loss of epithelial cell adhesion and polarity?
Interferon regulatory factor 3	Induction of interferon ß mRNA; transactivator of interferons	–	Inadequate cellular response to viral infection (no interference with viral replication, no increase of MHC-I, no activation of NK-cells)

Table 2 *continued* Cellular binding partners for E6

Cellular binding partner	Cellular function of the binding partner	Degradation (+/−)	Possible consequences of interaction for the cell
MAGI-1/2/3	Tight-junction proteins; complex formation with ß-catenin; regulation of PTEN tumour suppressor	+	Affecting Akt signalling?; p53-independent inhibition of apoptosis
Mcm7	DNA replication initiation and DNA replication licensing	+	Overriding the early G1-phase arrest point; modulation of Mcm7 abundance?
Mupp1	Multi PDZ scaffold protein; role in signal transduction?	+	Disruption of the assembly of signalling complexes at the epithelial cell membranes?
Paxillin	Focal adhesion protein; has a role in cell adhesion and regulation of the actin cytoskeleton	−	Disruption of the actin cytoskeleton and cell matrix interactions?
p53	Tumour suppressor protein; regulation of cell response to mitogenic events	+	Loss of cell-cycle control; anti-apoptotic effects
XRCC1	DNA repair protein	−	Interference with DNA repair efficiency

Table 3 Cellular binding partners for E7

Cellular binding partner	Cellular function of the binding partner	Possible consequences of interaction for the cell
Members of the AP1 family	Transcription factors	Transactivational abrogation of IRF-1 transcriptional activity
α-glucosidase	Glycolytic control enzyme	Allosterical activation resulting in depletion of intracellular glycogen stores; cell hyperproliferation promoted
CyclinA, cyclinE complexes	Kinase activity	Activation of cyclin A following activation of cyclin E
Histone H1 kinase	Kinase activity	Interference with G2/M transition of cell cycle?
hTid-1	Homologue of drosophila tumour suppressor protein Tid56 dnaJ protein, modulator of apoptosis	Activation of E2F-responsive promoters involved in J-domain function?
IGFBP-3 (insulin-like growth factor binding protein)	Transcriptional target of p53 limits cellular availability of IGFs (important for cellular survival)?	Decrease in amount of IGFBP
IRF-1 (interferon-γ-induced transcriptional factor)	Regulates expression of IFN-ß	Inhibition of the IRF-1-mediated activation of IFN-ß promoter by recruiting histone deacetylase to the promoter?
Mi2ß	Histone deacetylase	Abrogation of IRF-1 transcriptional activity
Mpp2	Forkhead transcription factor	Abrogation of IRF-1 transcriptional activity
M2 pyruvate kinase (M2-PK)	Modulation of the activity of glycolytic enzyme M2	Shifting the equilibrium from the high substrate-affinity tetrameric form to the low substrate-affinity dimeric state of M2-PK
pRb	Regulation of cell-cycle control via complex formation of E2F-transcription factors	Phosphorylation of pRb and subsequent release from E2F, ubiquitination and subsequent degradation
pRb-associated pocket proteins	Regulation of cell-cycle control	Loss of cell-cycle control and activation of specific genes for cell-cycle progression
p21 CIP-1	Cyclin-dependent kinase inhibitor	Growth stimulation via loss of cell-cycle control

Table 3 *continued* Cellular binding partners for E7

Cellular binding partner	Cellular function of the binding partner	Possible consequences of interaction for the cell
p27^{KIP-1}	Cyclin-dependent kinase inhibitor	Growth stimulation via loss of cell-cycle control
p48	Interferon regulatory protein (DNA-binding component of ISGF3); key messenger protein	Inhibition of interferon signal pathways via nuclear translocation of p48 upon IFN-α stimulation
Subunit4 ATPase	S4 subunit of the 26S-proteasome	pRB degradation via direct targeting to the proteasome?
TAF110 (TATA box-binding protein-associated factor)	Involved in initiation of transcription; coactivator in regulating transcription?	Modulation of transcription?
TATA box-binding protein	Involved in initiation of transcription	Interference with the activation of p53-responsive promoters?

As the details of these protein interactions are revealed, our knowledge of the differences between infection with HR and LR HPV genotypes will continue to expand.

Conclusions

- HPV genotypes are distinguished by DNA sequence differences within the coding regions of the early proteins, E6 and E7, and the late protein, L1

- The main HPV oncoproteins are E6 and E7

- The ability of anogenital E6 and E7 proteins to degrade cellular tumour suppressor proteins correlates with oncogenic potential

- This correlation has not been seen in cutaneous papillomaviruses

- A persistently HR HPV-infected cell undergoes continuous cell division and does not halt proliferation in response to DNA damage

References

1. Pfister H, Fuchs PG. Anatomy, taxonomy and evolution of papillomaviruses. *Intervirology* 1994;37:143–9

2. Orth G, Jablonska S, Breitburd F *et al*. The human papillomaviruses. *Bull Cancer* 1978;65:151–64

3. Bosch FX, Manos MM, Munoz N *et al*. Prevalence of human papillomavirus in cervical cancer: a worldwide perspective. International biological study on cervical cancer (IBSCC) Study Group. *J Natl Cancer Inst* 1995; 87:796–802

4. Bosch FX, Lorincz A, Munoz N *et al*. The causal relation between human papillomavirus and cervical cancer. *J Clin Pathol* 2002;55:244–65

5. zur Hausen H. Roots and perspectives of contemporary papillomavirus research. *J Cancer Res Clin Oncol* 1996;122:3–13

6. Walboomers JM, Jacobs MV, Manos MM *et al*. Human papillomavirus is a necessary cause of invasive cervical cancer worldwide. *J Pathol* 1999;189:12–9

7. Koutsky LA, Ault KA, Wheeler CM *et al*. A controlled trial of a human papillomavirus type 16 vaccine. *N Engl J Med* 2002;347:1645–51

8. Munoz N, Bosch FX, de Sanjose S *et al*. Epidemiologic classification of human papillomavirus types associated with cervical cancer. *N Engl J Med* 2003;348:518–27

9. Sedman SA, Barbosa MS, Vass WC *et al*. The full-length E6 protein of human papillomavirus type 16 has transforming and trans-activating activities and cooperates with E7 to immortalize keratinocytes in culture. *J Virol* 1991;65:4860–6

10. von Knebel Doeberitz M, Oltersdorf T, Schwarz E, Gissmann L. Correlation of modified human papilloma virus early gene expression with altered growth properties in C4-1 cervical carcinoma cells. *Cancer Res* 1988;48:3780–6

11. Halbert CL, Demers GW, Galloway DA. The E6 and E7 genes of human papillomavirus type 6 have weak immortalizing activity in human epithelial cells. *J Virol* 1992;66:2125–34

12. Munger K, Howley PM. Human papillomavirus immortalization and transformation functions. *Virus Res* 2002;89:213–28

13. Stubenrauch F, Laimins LA. Human papillomavirus life cycle: active and latent phases. *Semin Cancer Biol* 1999;9:379–86

14. Stubenrauch F, Zobel T, Iftner T. The E8 domain confers a novel long-distance transcriptional repression activity on the E8E2C protein of high-risk human papillomavirus type 31. *J Virol* 2001;75:4139–49

15. Hengstermann A, Linares LK, Ciechanover A *et al*. Complete switch from Mdm2 to human papillomavirus E6-mediated degradation of p53 in cervical cancer cells. *Proc Natl Acad Sci USA* 2001;98:1218–23

16. Huibregtse JM, Scheffner M, Howley PM. A cellular protein mediates association of p53 with the E6 oncoprotein of human papillomavirus types 16 or 18. *EMBO J* 1991;10:4129–35

17. Mantovani F, Banks L. The human papillomavirus E6 protein and its contribution to malignant progression. *Oncogene* 2001;20:7874–87

18. Scheffner M, Werness BA, Huibregtse JM *et al*. The E6 oncoprotein encoded by human papillomavirus types 16 and 18 promotes the degradation of p53. *Cell* 1990;63:1129–36

19. Quint WG, Scholte G, van Doorn LJ *et al*. Comparative analysis of human papillomavirus infections in cervical scrapes and biopsy specimens by general SPF(10) PCR and HPV genotyping. *J Pathol* 2001;194:51–8

20. Werness BA, Levine AJ, Howley PM. Association of human papillomavirus types 16 and 18 E6 proteins with p53. *Science* 1990;248:76–9

21. Boyer SN, Wazer DE, Band V. E7 protein of human papilloma virus-16 induces degradation of retinoblastoma protein through the ubiquitin-proteasome pathway. *Cancer Res* 1996;56:4620–4

22. Munger K, Basile JR, Duensing S *et al*. Biological activities and molecular targets of the human papillomavirus E7 oncoprotein. *Oncogene* 2001;20:7888–98

23. Funk JO, Waga S, Harry JB *et al*. Inhibition of CDK activity and PCNA-dependent DNA replication by p21 is blocked by interaction with the HPV-16 E7 oncoprotein. *Genes Dev* 1997;11:2090–100

24. Iftner T, Elbel M, Schopp B *et al*. Interference of papillomavirus E6 protein with single-strand break repair by interaction with XRCC1. *EMBO J* 2002;21:4741–8

2. Human papillomavirus and genital warts: relationship and management

Fiona Lyons

- The natural history of genital warts is generally benign and the human papillomavirus (HPV) types responsible for genital warts (e.g. 6 and 11) are not the same types that are associated with an increased risk for cervical cancer development

- Spontaneous resolution of genital warts occurs in 10–20% of cases

- All treatment options have an associated failure rate, and recurrence of genital warts after treatment is common

- Any condition producing impaired cell-mediated immunity in HPV-infected individuals is likely to increase disease expression, decrease response to treatment and increase relapse rates

- Condoms have not been shown to reduce transmission of HPV

Introduction

Genital warts are caused by certain types of human papillomavirus (HPV), although these types are different from those associated with an increased risk of cervical cancer development. Infection is common amongst sexually active adults and acquisition is usually sexual. The incubation period from time of infection to development of genital warts is highly variable, although many infected individuals will never develop them.

Prevalence of HPV and genital warts

The burden of disease caused by HPV is substantial. Estimates of prevalence indicate that, worldwide, 15% of the adult population have a current HPV infection and 1% have genital warts.[1] In 1994, the US Institute of Medicine estimated that the total annual cost of HPV-related disease was $3827 million, excluding HPV-related cancer.[2] Between 1972 and 2002, the number of all genital wart diagnoses (first episode, recurrent and re-registered cases), at genitourinary medicine clinics in the UK, increased more than 6-fold in men and 10-fold in women.[3]

Factors associated with the acquisition of HPV infection

The risk of acquiring HPV infection in females has been shown to increase with cigarette smoking, oral contraceptive use and intercourse with a new male partner.[4] The same study reported that infection in virgins was rare, although any type of non-penetrative sexual contact was associated with an increased risk, suggesting that this is a plausible route of HPV acquisition in virgins.[4]

Studies on the potential benefit of condom use in preventing HPV infection have been inconclusive. A recent meta-analysis suggests that condoms may not prevent HPV infection, but may reduce the risk of genital warts, high-grade cervical intraepithelial neoplasia (CIN) and invasive cancer.[5] The authors pointed out, however, that the data are too inconsistent to provide precise risk estimates. The use of condoms remains strongly recommended, since it reduces the transmission of other sexually transmitted infections (STIs), such as human immunodeficiency virus (HIV) and chlamydia.

Factors associated with expression of HPV disease

Any situation where there is a deficiency of cell-mediated immunity will increase the likelihood of HPV disease expression. Therefore, subsequent to HPV exposure, transplant recipients, patients with diabetes mellitus or HIV, or those on immunosuppressant drugs, such as steroids and chemotherapy, are more likely to develop HPV disease, including genital warts.[6] Cigarette smoking also reduces cell-mediated immunity and there is a correlation between smoking and malignant manifestations of HPV disease.[7]

Genital warts and HPV types

Over 130 HPV types have been identified and about 40 of these can infect the genital tract. More than 90% of genital wart lesions examined are associated with HPV types 6 and 11. A recently published study of the epidemiology of HPV types found that these types (6 and 11) are associated with a low potential risk for the development of malignancy.[8]

Development of genital warts

Micro-abrasions in the skin surface allow the entry of HPV. Stratified squamous epithelial cells (keratinocytes) become infected with HPV and the virus then spreads to the deep basal layers of the epithelium. Following infection with HPV, the virus stimulates the growth of the infected keratinocytes. HPV-induced cell growth causes the accumulation of infected cells that become recognized as a wart.

In the deep basal layers of the epithelium there is little HPV replication, no cell lysis and, therefore, little exposure of the antigen (HPV) to the immune system. Furthermore, the virus does not kill HPV-infected cells, so there is no local inflammation, no release of local cytokines, no antigen-presenting cell activation and no cell-mediated immune response. The host remains immune ignorant, with the consequence that HPV can be present for long periods of time. It is only during the process of desquamation of mature cells that large numbers of viruses are shed. The progeny of a single HPV-infected cell may extend over 2–3 mm^2 of skin.[9] In order to eradicate HPV, virus must be exposed to the immune system, which occurs spontaneously in 10–20% of patients. The trigger for this exposure is not known, but biopsies from patients who have experienced spontaneous resolution of warts show an increased production of cytokines such as IFN and IL-12.

Clinical features

Symptoms

Genital warts (Figures 1a and b) may cause irritation and soreness, particularly in the perianal region, and although the majority cause little physical discomfort, the infection is psychologically distressing to many people affected.[10]

Signs

Warts may occur singly, or may be multiple, occurring in clusters or as plaques. They can be flat, dome-shaped, keratotic, pedunculated or cauliflower-shaped. Warts on warm, moist, non-hair-bearing skin tend to be soft and non-keratinized, while those on dry, hairy skin tend to be firm and keratinized. Warts can occur both externally and internally in the genital area, and extragenital warts can occur on the face and in the oral cavity.

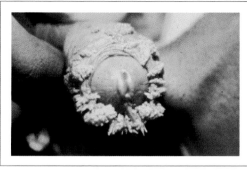
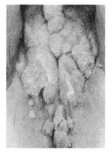

Figure 1a Penile wart   **Figure 1b** Vulval wart

Diagnosis

Diagnosis is clinical, from a naked-eye examination in the majority of cases. Biopsy is not routinely recommended, but can be useful if the diagnosis is in doubt or if the features are atypical.

Differential diagnoses

- Condyloma lata (secondary syphilis)
- Molluscum contagiosum (caused by pox virus)
- Dysplastic and benign nevi
- Invasive cancers
- In males: pearly papules that occur around the coronal sulcus

Management

Cervical cytology in women with genital warts

The UK National Health Service Cervical Screening Programme recommends that no change of screening interval in women with anogenital warts is needed.[11] Similarly, US guidelines recommend that the frequency of screening does not need to be increased in women with genital warts.[12] For women presenting with genital warts who are below the recommended age for commencement of cervical screening, it is *not* necessary to perform cervical screening until they have reached the appropriate age.

STI screening and sexual partners

An STI screen is recommended, as many patients will have concurrent infections.[13] Sexual partners do not need to be contact traced but may benefit from a clinical assessment, as they may have undetected genital warts or other STIs.

Treatment

Since the virus can be present in skin of normal appearance, all treatments that eradicate wart tissue have significant failure and relapse rates. Without treatment, spontaneous resolution of genital warts will occur in 10–20% of individuals, so non-treatment is an option at any site, particularly for warts in the vagina or anal canal. Standardized treatment protocols and algorithms used at clinics have been shown to improve treatment success.[14] Treatment choice depends on the morphology, number and distribution of warts. Soft non-keratinized warts respond well to podophyllin, podophyllotoxin and trichloroacetic acid. Keratinized lesions are better treated with physical ablative methods such as cryotherapy, excision or electrocautery.[15] Imiquimod may be suitable for both types. Patients with a small number of minor warts are best treated with ablative therapy from the outset, irrespective of type.

Chemical applications

Podophyllotoxin

Podophyllotoxin is a purified extract of the non-standardized cytotoxic compound podophyllin, devoid of the mutagenic flavonoids quercetin and kaempherol. It is superior to, and has largely replaced, podophyllin,[16] which was associated with severe local reactions, and, if incorrectly applied, with serious adverse systemic events.[17] Animal studies have demonstrated teratogenic and oncogenic potential with podophyllin,[18,19] which should, therefore, be avoided for use on the cervix or in the anal canal, and in pregnancy. Furthermore, clinical studies have demonstrated the inferior efficacy of podophyllin, compared with podophyllotoxin.

Podophyllotoxin is available in the form of a 0.5% solution or as a 0.15% cream and, unlike podophyllin, is suitable for home treatment. Treatment cycles consist of twice-daily application for 3 days, followed by 4 days' rest. This is repeated for 2–4 cycles. The cream may be easier for many patients to apply, especially on the perianal skin. Common side-effects include local irritation and inflammation, which may require treatment interruption, but rarely cessation. The safety of podophyllotoxin in pregnancy has not been established and use in pregnancy is not recommended.

Trichloroacetic acid

Trichloroacetic acid (TCA) 80–90% solution is suitable for weekly application in a specialist clinic setting only. Its effectiveness in clinical trials ranges from 63% to 70%, and does not exceed that for cryotherapy or laser therapy.[12] This agent is probably most effective for treating small residual warts, often after a period of treatment with podophyllotoxin or cryotherapy. TCA can be used at most anatomical sites, but is caustic to both skin and mucous membranes, resulting in cellular necrosis. Overapplication can result in TCA spreading onto adjacent, unaffected skin, leading to the damage and sometimes ulceration of healthy skin. Careful application, with allowance for a sufficient drying time, reduces this problem. A neutralizing agent, such as sodium bicarbonate, should always be available in case of excess application or spills.

Imiquimod

Imiquimod is an immune-response modifier which does not have any *in vitro* antiviral activity. It is available as a 5% cream for home-based therapy, and is suitable for use on all external genital warts, but is not recommended for internal use or in pregnancy. Its use in uncircumcised men has been shown to be safe.[20] The cream is applied to lesions three times weekly (for up to 16 weeks) and washed off 6–10 hours later. Response to treatment may be delayed for several weeks. Mild local erythema is common and can occasionally be severe, necessitating termination of treatment. High patient satisfaction has been reported with imiquimod cream.[21]

5-Fluorouracil

5-Fluorouracil is a DNA antimetabolite, available in a 5% cream, but its use is limited by severe local side-effects. It may be teratogenic, so should not be used in pregnancy. This agent is rarely used and, since satisfactory alternatives exist, the treatment is no longer recommended unless expert advice is available.[11]

Interferons

Various regimens have been described that utilize interferons alpha, beta and gamma as creams, or as intralesional or systemic injections. Clinical utility is limited by expense, systemic side-effects and a variable response rate. Interferons should not be used routinely for the treatment of genital warts.

Physical ablation

Cryotherapy

The application of a liquid nitrogen spray or a cryoprobe causes cytolysis at the dermal epidermal junction, resulting in necrosis of genital warts. Several days after treatment, the treated area sloughs, inflammation ensues and healing subsequently occurs. Treatment should be applied until a 'halo' of a few millimetres in size appears around the treated area, which is then allowed to thaw before refreezing with more liquid nitrogen.

Excision

Surgical removal of warts can be undertaken with local anaesthetic injection or under general anaesthetic. Removal of warts under local anaesthetic injection has been reported to be a good method of treatment for small numbers of warts and is probably underutilized.[22] Haemostasis can be established using electrosurgery or by the application of a haemostatic solution such as silver nitrate. For extensive anogenital warts, treatment by excision under general anaesthetic may need to be carried out over more than one treatment session. A recent audit of surgical excision found that it was acceptable to patients and had a recurrence rate of 24% at 6 months.[23] The utility of combined treatment with surgery and imiquimod is currently under investigation.

Electrosurgery

Electrosurgical techniques include electrocautery and electro-fulguration. Skin bridges between treatment sites facilitate healing and minimize scarring. It is important to note that with all surgical and laser techniques, the early response rates suggest superiority over other non-surgical techniques. However, this superiority usually disappears at 3 months of follow-up, reflecting the time required for non-surgical techniques to work.

Laser treatment

The carbon dioxide laser is especially suitable for large-volume warts and can be used at difficult anatomical sites, such as the urethral meatus, or intra-anally.[24] It is an expensive treatment option with variable response rates. Electrosurgical and laser techniques produce a plume of smoke, which has been shown to contain HPV DNA, and may potentially cause infection of the respiratory tract in operating personnel. It is essential, therefore, that masks be worn and adequate extraction provided during these procedures.[25]

Treatment according to wart location

Treatment options according to wart location are presented in Table 1. For intravaginal warts, withholding treatment should be considered, particularly in pregnancy, since warts will often spontaneously regress after delivery. The use of imiquimod on external genital warts may simultaneously confer some therapeutic benefit to internal genital warts. Although there is little information to indicate the best practice for the management of cervical genital warts, some evidence supports the use of colposcopically directed biopsy to establish a histological diagnosis before treatment decisions are made.[26] However, this practice runs the risk of over-screening and over-treatment, particularly in younger women. If histology shows no evidence of CIN, then cryotherapy, electrosurgery or TCA may be used.

For warts involving the urethral meatus, if the base of the lesion is seen, treatment options are as shown in Table 1. Cases lying deeper in the urethra should be referred for urological assessment and management.

Table 1 Treatment options according to wart location

Treatment	Wart location			
	Intravaginal	Cervix	Urethral meatus	Intra-anal
Surgical removal	✓	✓	✓	✓
Cryotherapy	✓	✓	✓	✓
Electrosurgery	✓	✓	✓	✓
Trichloroacetic acid	✓	✓	✓	✓
Imiquimod	✓		✓	
Podophyllotoxin		✓	✓	
Laser				✓

Genital warts in pregnancy

Genital warts in pregnancy can cause great anxiety in women who fear that they may pass the virus to their baby during labour and delivery. Safe treatment options include cryotherapy, TCA application or surgery. Podophyllin, podophyllotoxin and 5-fluorouracil are contraindicated because of possible teratogenic effects, and imiquimod is not approved for use in pregnancy. Following vertical exposure to HPV, potential problems for the infant are the development of laryngeal papillomatosis and anogenital warts. Very rarely, a Caesarean section is indicated where there is blockage of the vaginal outlet with warts or the presence of gross cervical warts.

Conclusions

- HPV types causing genital warts are different from those associated with an increased risk of developing cervical cancer

- Treatment choice depends on the morphology, number and site distribution of warts

- All treatment options are prone to result in relapse

References

1. Koutsky LA, Galloway DA, Holmes KK. Epidemiology of genital human papillomavirus infection. *Epidemiol Rev* 1988;10:122–63

2. Eng TR, Butler WT. The neglected health and economic impact of STD's, The hidden epidemic: confronting sexually transmitted diseases, Committee on Prevention and Control of Sexually Transmitted Disease, Institute of Medicine, National Academic Press, 1997, pp 28–68

3. www.hpa.org.uk/infections/topics_az/hiv_and_sti/sti-warts/epidemiology/epidemiology.htm. Health Protection Agency Guidelines. Date acccessed, 23 July 2004

4. Winer RL, Lee SK, Hughes JP *et al*. Genital human papillomavirus infection: incidence and risk factors in a cohort of female university students. *Am J Epidemiol* 2003;157:218–26

5. Manhart LE, Koutsky LA. Do condoms prevent genital HPV infection, external genital warts, or cervical neoplasia? A meta-analysis. S*ex Transm Dis* 2002;29:725–35

6. Kataja V, Syrjanen S, Yliskoski M *et al*. Risk factors associated with cervical human papillomavirus infections: a case-control study. *Am J Epidemiol* 1993;138:735–45

7. Feldman JG, Chirgwin K, Dehovitz JA, Minkoff H. The association of smoking and risk of condyloma acuminatum in women. *Obstet Gynecol* 1997;89:346–50

8. Munoz N, Bosch FX, de Sanjose S *et al*. Epidemiologic classification of human papillomavirus types associated with cervical cancer. *N Engl J Med* 2003;348:518–27

9. Steele JC, Gallimore PH. Humoral assays of human sera to disrupted and nondisrupted epitopes of human papillomavirus type 1. *Virology* 1990; 174:388–98

10. Clarke P, Ebel C, Catotti DN, Stewart S. The psychosocial impact of human papillomavirus infection: implications for health care providers. *Int J STD AIDS* 1996;7:197–200

11. Clinical Effectiveness Guidelines; British Association for Sexual Health and HIV. National guidelines for the management of anogenital warts. www.mssvd.org.uk, 2002. Date acccessed, 23 July 2004

12. Wiley D, Douglas J, Beutner K. External genital warts: diagnosis treatment and prevention. *Clin Infect Diseases* 2002;35(Suppl 2):s210–24

13. Pakianathan MR, Ross JD, McMillan A. Characterizing patients with multiple sexually acquired infections: a multivariate analysis. *Int J STD AIDS* 1996;7:359–61

14. Reynold M, Fraser P, Lacey C. Audits of the treatment of genital warts; closing the feedback loop. *Int J STD AIDS* 1996;7:347–52

15. Eron LJ. Human papillomaviruses and anogenital disease, in Gorbach SL, Bartlett JG, Blacklow NR (eds): Infectious diseases. Philadelphia, WE Saunders, 1992, pp 952–6

16. Kinghorn GR, McMillan A, Mulcahy F *et al*. An open, comparative, study of the efficacy of 0.5% podophyllotoxin lotion and 25% podophyllotoxin solution in the treatment of condylomata acuminata in males and females. *Int J STD AIDS* 1993;4:194–9

17. Marcus J, Camisa C. Podophyllin therapy for condyloma acuminatum. *Int J Dermatol* 1990;29:693–8

18. Sabine JR, Horton BJ, Wicks MB. Spontaneous tumors in C3H-A vy and C3H-A vy fB mice: high incidence in the United States and low incidence in Australia. *J Natl Cancer Inst* 1973;50:1237–42

19. Kaminetski HA, Swerdiow M. Podophyllin and the mouse cervix. *Am J Obstet Gynecol* 1965;93:486–90

20. Gollnick H, Barasso R, Jappe U *et al*. Safety and efficacy of imiquimod 5% cream in the treatment of penile genital warts in uncircumcised men when applied three times weekly or once per day. *Int J STD AIDS* 2001;12:22–8

21. O'Mahony C, Law C, Gollnick HP, Marini M. New patient-applied therapy for anogenital warts is rated favourably by patients. *Int J STD AIDS* 2001; 12:565–70

22. Bonnez W, Oakes D, Choi A *et al*. Therapeutic efficacy and complications of excisional biopsy of condyloma acuminatum. *Sex Transm Dis* 1996; 23:273–6

23. Chancellor R, Alexander I. A five-year audit of the treatment of extensive anogenital warts by day case electrosurgery under general anaesthesia. *Int J STD AIDS* 2002;13:786–9

24. Ferenczy A. Laser treatment of genital condylomata acuminata. *Obstet Gynecol* 1984;63:703–7

25. Ferenczy A, Bergeron C, Richart RM. Human papillomavirus DNA in CO2 laser-generated plume of smoke and its consequences to the surgeon. *Obstet Gynecol* 1990;75:114–8

26. Murphy M, Fairley I, Wilson J. Exophytic cervical warts – an indication for colposcopy? *Genitourin Med* 1993;69:81–2

3. Understanding the origin of cervical cancer

*F Xavier Bosch, Sílvia de Sanjosé and
Xavier Castellsagué*

- Human papillomavirus (HPV) infections are among the most common sexually transmitted infections

- Sexually transmitted infection of high-risk (HR) HPV precedes cervical cancer development by several years

- Persistence of an HR HPV type is a necessary causal factor for invasive cervical disease

- The definition of HR types is being refined by genotyping and by ongoing epidemiological investigations in distinct populations

- Steroid hormones and tobacco smoking interact with HPV in the neoplastic process

Introduction

The discovery that cervical cancer is a rare consequence of a common infection is as momentous for public health as the demonstration of the association between cigarette smoking and lung cancer. Infection with some mucosal types of human papillomavirus (HPV) is now known to precede cervical cancer development by several years. Many studies have shown unequivocally that HPV DNA can be detected in ≥99.7% of adequate cervical cancer specimens, compared with 5–20% of cervical specimens from women identified as suitable epidemiological controls.[1–3] HPV has been recognized as a prerequisite for cervical cancer, and certain types of HPV have now been designated as the first ever identified *necessary cause* of a human cancer.

Natural history of HPV infections

HPV infections are among the most common sexually transmitted infections in most populations, and estimates of exposure range from 15–20% in many European countries to 70% in the US or 95% in high-risk populations in Africa.[4]

Both the prevalence of HPV DNA in cervical cells and the prevalence of cervical cancer in the population are closely related to the age of subjects, although the age profiles differ. HPV infections are highly prevalent in young individuals, whereas invasive cervical cancer does not typically develop until the third decade of life or later. Figure 1 shows the age-specific prevalence of high-risk (HR) HPV DNA in a screening programme and the corresponding age-specific incidence rates (ASIR) of cervical cancer in The Netherlands (adapted from Bosch *et al.*, 2002).[3]

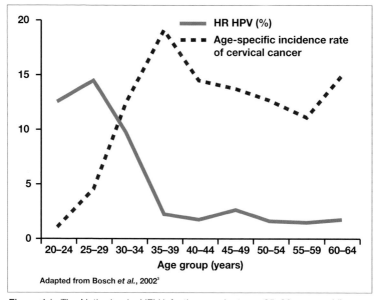

Adapted from Bosch et al., 2002[3]

Figure 1 In The Netherlands, HPV infections peak at age 25–30 years, while cervical cancer peaks after age 40 years

Understanding the origin of cervical cancer

Similar age-related prevalence rates are found across other settings and in countries with both high and low incidences of cervical cancer. The cross-sectional prevalence of HPV DNA decreases spontaneously to a background level of 2–8% in most populations in the age group of 30 years and above. In countries where there is intensive screening of young women, part of the HPV prevalence reduction could be attributable to aggressive treatment of HPV-related cervical lesions. Women who remain chronic HPV carriers are now recognized as the true high-risk group for cervical cancer. In some populations, a second peak of HPV DNA prevalence has been observed for older women (age group ≥50 years), although the significance of this peak in relation to the risk of cervical cancer in these older age groups is still unknown.

Most HPV exposure occurs soon after sexual initiation. Assessment of virgins after their sexual debut showed that exposure levels to HPV were 40% after 24 months, and 70% by 56 months.[5]

Key determinants of HPV prevalence among women

- Number of sexual partners
- Age at which sexual intercourse was initiated
- Likelihood that each of her sexual partners was an HPV carrier

---

Duration of HPV infection

In follow-up studies of women, repeated sampling for viral persistence and cervical abnormalities have shown that median durations of infection are longer for HR HPV types, compared with those for low-risk (LR) HPV types (8.0–13.5 vs 4.8–8.2 months, respectively),[6–8] and the longest persistence occurs with type 16. However, the time intervals determined in all these studies may still be inaccurate, because of imprecise estimates of the time of first exposure; variability in the definition of endpoints; and censoring due to treatment of early lesions.

The vector role of male partners

Studies using questionnaires have addressed the role of sexual behaviour of the husbands or sexual partners of cervical cancer cases in disease transmission, while more recent investigations have also tested for HPV DNA in exfoliated cells from the penile shaft, the coronal sulcus and the distal urethra. Such studies have consistently shown that the risk of developing cervical cancer for a woman is predicted as much by the sexual behaviour of her partner as by her own sexual behaviour. In populations where female monogamy is dominant, female sex workers have an important influence on the maintenance and transmission of HPV infections. More recently, it has been possible to confirm that male circumcision protects males from becoming HPV carriers, and consequently protects their wives from developing cervical cancer.[9] These studies provide a virological basis for clinical observations that have led to the scientific hypothesis that male sexual behaviour is a central determinant of the incidence of cervical cancer.

From HPV infection to abnormal cervical cytology

Follow-up studies of women with and without cervical abnormalities have indicated that persistence of HR HPV infection is necessary for the development, maintenance and progression of cervical intraepithelial neoplasia (CIN).[10] A substantial proportion of women (15–30%) with HR HPV DNA, who are cytomorphologically normal at recruitment, will develop CIN 2 or CIN 3 within the 4-year interval following the identification of infection.[11] Conversely, among women with equivocal or low-grade dysplasia who are HPV-negative, the majority will become cytologically negative over the following 2 years. Women who test positive for LR HPVs rarely become persistent carriers and their probability of progression to CIN 2–3 is extremely low.[12,13]

Table 1 Progression from HPV infection to HSIL/CIN 2–3

Normal cytology	Progression to HSIL/CIN 2–3 (%)	Relative risk for progression (HPV+ vs HPV–)	Reference
HPV+ HPV–	7 0.1	NA	11
HPV+[a] HPV–[a]	8.7[b] 0.7[b]	12.3 (2.6–57.5)	14
HPV+	NA	7.8 (2.7–22.0)	8
HPV+[a]	NA	20.9 (8.6–51.0)	7
HPV+ (16 or 18) HPV–	28 3	11 (8.6–51.0)	15

[a]Two consecutive tests; [b]per 100 woman-months; HSIL: High-grade squamous intra-epithelial lesion

The results of several studies comparing the progression rate of women with normal cytology to high-grade squamous intraepithelial lesions (HSIL) as a function of their HPV DNA status at recruitment are summarized in Table 1. Such studies indicate an increased relative risk (RR) in patients who test HPV-positive, compared with those who test negative, particularly when two consecutive tests are performed. Furthermore, recent evidence suggests that clearance of HR HPV is associated with regression of existing CIN lesions.[12]

Cross-protection following type-specific infection

Data from an interesting study, reporting on the likelihood of developing a second type-specific HPV infection following a primary infection,[16] suggests that, after resolving one infection, women are protected against re-infection with the same HPV type but not against other types – even those closely related. This observation complicates the interpretation of follow-up studies, and the definition of persistence. Studies investigating HPV transmission or natural history clearly benefit from the use of type-specific HPV testing systems.

Criteria to support causality of viral exposure for cervical cancer

Criteria to support epidemiological evidence for HPV as a cause of human cancer have been evaluated, and several have been widely adopted (for a review, see Bosch et al., 2002[3]).

HPV infection precedes the development of cervical cancer

The bulk of HPV infections precede the bulk of cervical cancer by two to three decades (Figure 1) and support a link between prior exposure and disease. However, follow-up studies are ethically constrained to intervene at the stage of pre-invasive disease (CIN 2 and above in most

> ## Key supportive criteria
>
> - HPV infection must precede the development of cervical cancer
>
> - Association between HPV infection and cervical cancer must be strong and consistent:
>   - Strength is measured by the odds ratio (OR) or RR in studies comparing cancer risk between HPV+ and HPV– women
>   - Consistency is shown by similar results from studies with different settings, different observers, and different methods for study design and HPV testing
> - Proposed biological mechanisms must be consistent with existing knowledge

settings), so the evolution of the HPV infection to invasive cancer cannot be directly assessed in prospective studies. Retrospective studies on archival Papanicolaou (Pap) cervical smear samples have successfully documented the existence of HPV exposure decades before the development of the disease, and have shown RR estimates for HPV positivity and invasive cervical cancer of 16.4 (95% confidence interval [CI]: 4.4–75.1) and 32 (95% CI: 6.8–153), respectively.[13]

Strong and consistent association between HPV infection and cervical cancer

The prevalence of HPV DNA in a series of case–control studies consistently shows proportions of viral DNA in 85–95% of cases, compared with 5–15% in epidemiologically matched controls. Reported data have shown an increased prevalence, from 75% to approximately 95%, since outdated, less sensitive PCR detection systems (MYO9/11 PCR) have been replaced by more sensitive systems (GP5+/6+, PGMY09/11). Estimates of odds ratios (ORs) for the development of cervical cancer in individuals infected with any

HR HPV range from 50 to 100, and ORs for specific associations (e.g. HPV 16 and squamous cell cancer, and HPV 18 and cervical adenocarcinomas) range from 100 to 900. These OR estimates allow consistent calculations of attributable fractions (AFs) – the proportion of cervical cancer that can be attributed to HR HPV infection – which lie in the range 90–95%, in all geographical populations. These studies also demonstrate consistent similarities between squamous cell carcinomas and adenocarcinomas, between pre-invasive disease and invasive cancer, and between risk estimates for HPV DNA (all types considered) and risk estimates restricted to HR types (reviewed in Bosch et al., 2002[3]).

Given the case–control design of these studies, these ORs reflect the risk in relation to existing HPV DNA infection (HPV DNA point prevalence), but not in relation to the cumulative lifetime exposure, a parameter that is obviously difficult to study. It is customary to interpret the HPV DNA point prevalence at ages 40 years and above as a reflection of viral persistence. However, much research is still required to accurately define viral persistence and clarify its relevance in the application of HPV testing for screening and patient management.

Results from a multicentre study conducted by the International Agency for Research on Cancer (IARC), using genotyping in 1545 women with cervical cancer, have provided type-specific estimates of genotype prevalence and OR data (Figure 2).[17]

The most common HPV types may have some selective advantage for transmission and/or establishing persistent infections. Prevalence and OR data also indicate that HPVs 31, 33, 35, 45, 51, 52, 56, 58, 59, 68, 73 and 82 should be considered, in addition to HPV 16 and HPV 18, as human carcinogens.[17]

The prevalence of multiple HPV types in single cervical specimens varies widely, according to the study population. Populations with high-risk sexual behaviour (e.g. prostitutes) or HIV seropositivity show consistently higher rates of multiple infections. However, studies that have compared risk estimates in women tend to show that multiple infections do not convey a statistically significantly increased risk over single infections.

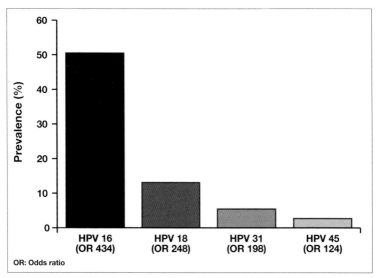

Figure 2 Prevalence of the four most common HPV types in cervical cancer, and risk estimates for squamous cell carcinomas (IARC results)[17]

HPV infection provides biological plausibility and coherence with previous knowledge

Viral and host interactions leading to cell transformation and malignancy have been described (see Chapter 1) which are in accordance with known mechanisms of carcinogenesis (Figure 3).

Other relevant factors in cervical carcinogenesis

Most of the sexual behaviour parameters previously linked to the development of cervical cancer have been shown to be surrogate measures of HPV exposure. Other factors associated with an increased risk of cervical cancer – oral contraceptive (OC) use, parity and smoking – are shown in Table 2.

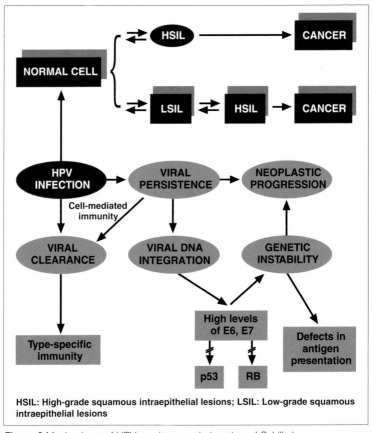

Figure 3 Mechanisms of HPV carcinogenesis (courtesy J Schiller)

In the IARC's multicentre case–control study, OC use was associated with a significant increase in risk, which was strongly related to length of use. The OR was 2.72 (95% CI: 1.36–5.46) for 5–9 years of use and 4.48 (95% CI: 2.24–9.36) for 10+ years of use.[18] However, subgroup analyses in other studies have reported no or only weak associations between OC use and cervical cancer.[19] These apparently conflicting results may reflect the increased cytological surveillance of women who are using OCs in developed countries, and the use of different

Table 2 Environmental risk factors in HPV carcinogenesis

Risk factor	Odds ratio (95% CI)	Reference
Oral contraceptive (OC) use		
HPV+, OC+ HPV+, OC–	1.47 (1.02–2.12)	18
Parity		
HPV+, > 7 births HPV+, 0 births	3.8 (2.7–5.5)	20
HPV+, > 7 births HPV+, 1–2 births	2.3 (1.6–3.2)	20
Smoking		
HPV+, current smoker	2.3	21

case definitions in cohort studies (atypical squamous cells of undetermined significance to HSIL/CIN 3) in contrast to case–control studies (cervical cancer). A recent meta-analysis confirmed the interaction between OC use and HPV exposure, particularly for prolonged periods, in relation to the risk of cervical cancer.[22]

The IARC studies also identified high parity as a risk factor (Table 2),[20] and similar results were obtained in Costa Rica[23] and in Thailand.[19] These findings strongly suggest that steroid hormones interact with HPV in the neoplastic process.

Smoking cigarettes is a universal cofactor for cervical cancer among HPV-positive women.[24]

Conclusions

- Natural history studies of HPV infections are able to explain, in virological terms, most of the observations that have historically linked HPV to cervical cancer

- Women who remain chronic HPV carriers are now recognized as the true high-risk group for cervical cancer

- Other factors implicated as causal agents are: long-term OC use, the high number of full-term pregnancies and smoking. In the absence of HPV DNA, it is uncertain if these co-factors increase the risk of cervical cancer

- HPV testing with HR cocktails are sufficient for screening programmes and clinical management. Investigations of HPV transmission or natural history clearly benefit from the use of type-specific HPV testing systems

- Public health institutions can now evaluate these advances, consider the costs and benefits involved, and apply this knowledge to their guidelines, recommendations and policy

References

1. Walboomers JM, Jacobs MV, Manos MM et al. Human papillomavirus is a necessary cause of invasive cervical cancer worldwide. J Pathol 1999;189:12–9

2. Bosch FX, Manos MM, Munoz N et al. Prevalence of human papillomavirus in cervical cancer: a worldwide perspective. International biological study on cervical cancer (IBSCC) Study Group. J Natl Cancer Inst 1995; 87:796–802

3. Bosch FX, Lorincz A, Munoz N et al. The causal relation between human papillomavirus and cervical cancer. J Clin Pathol 2002;55:244–65

4. Bosch FX, de Sanjose S. Human papillomavirus and cervical cancer – burden and assessment of causality. J Natl Cancer Inst Monogr 2003:3–13

5. Winer RL, Lee SK, Hughes JP et al. Genital human papillomavirus infection: incidence and risk factors in a cohort of female university students. Am J Epidemiol 2003;157:218–26

6. Franco EL, Villa LL, Sobrinho JP et al. Epidemiology of acquisition and clearance of cervical human papillomavirus infection in women from a high-risk area for cervical cancer. J Infect Dis 1999;180:1415–23

7. Ho GY, Bierman R, Beardsley L et al. Natural history of cervicovaginal papillomavirus infection in young women. N Engl J Med 1998;338:423–8

8. Woodman CB, Collins S, Winter H et al. Natural history of cervical human papillomavirus infection in young women: a longitudinal cohort study. Lancet 2001;357:1831–6

9. Castellsague X, Bosch FX, Munoz N et al. Male circumcision, penile human papillomavirus infection, and cervical cancer in female partners. N Engl J Med 2002;346:1105–12

10. Nobbenhuis MA, Walboomers JM, Helmerhorst TJ et al. Relation of human papillomavirus status to cervical lesions and consequences for cervical-cancer screening: a prospective study. Lancet 1999;354:20–5

11. Rozendaal L, Walboomers JM, van der Linden JC et al. PCR-based high-risk HPV test in cervical cancer screening gives objective risk assessment of women with cytomorphologically normal cervical smears. Int J Cancer 1996;68:766–9

12. Nobbenhuis MA, Helmerhorst TJ, van den Brule AJ et al. Cytological regression and clearance of high-risk human papillomavirus in women with an abnormal cervical smear. Lancet 2001;358:1782–3

13. Zielinski GD, Snijders PJ, Rozendaal L *et al*. HPV presence precedes abnormal cytology in women developing cervical cancer and signals false negative smears. *Br J Cancer* 2001;85:398–404

14. Schlecht NF, Kulaga S, Robitaille J *et al*. Persistent human papillomavirus infection as a predictor of cervical intraepithelial neoplasia. *JAMA* 2001;286:3106–14

15. Koutsky LA, Holmes KK, Critchlow CW *et al*. A cohort study of the risk of cervical intraepithelial neoplasia grade 2 or 3 in relation to papillomavirus infection. *N Engl J Med* 1992;327:1272–8

16. Thomas KK, Hughes JP, Kuypers JM *et al*. Concurrent and sequential acquisition of different genital human papillomavirus types. *J Infect Dis* 2000;182:1097–102

17. Munoz N, Bosch FX, de Sanjose S *et al*. Epidemiologic classification of human papillomavirus types associated with cervical cancer. *N Engl J Med* 2003;348:518–27

18. Moreno V, Bosch FX, Munoz N *et al*. Effect of oral contraceptives on risk of cervical cancer in women with human papillomavirus infection: the IARC multicentric case-control study. *Lancet* 2002;359:1085–92

19. Thomas DB, Ray RM, Koetsawang A *et al*. Human papillomaviruses and cervical cancer in Bangkok. I. Risk factors for invasive cervical carcinomas with human papillomavirus types 16 and 18 DNA. *Am J Epidemiol* 2001;153:723–31

20. Munoz N, Franceschi S, Bosetti C *et al*. Role of parity and human papillomavirus in cervical cancer: the IARC multicentric case-control study. *Lancet* 2002;359:1093–101

21. Plummer M, Herrero R, Franceschi S *et al*. Smoking and cervical cancer: pooled analysis of the IARC multi-centric case-control study. *Cancer Causes Control* 2003;14:805–14

22. Smith JS, Green J, Berrington de Gonzalez A *et al*. Cervical cancer and use of hormonal contraceptives: a systematic review. *Lancet* 2003;361:1159–67

23. Hildesheim A, Herrero R, Castle PE *et al*. HPV co-factors related to the development of cervical cancer: results from a population-based study in Costa Rica. *Br J Cancer* 2001;84:1219–26

24. Castellsague X, Munoz N. Cofactors in human papillomavirus carcinogenesis – role of parity, oral contraceptives and tobacco smoking. *J Natl Cancer Inst Monogr* 2003;20–8

4. Viral treatment and prophylactic vaccination strategies

Toli S Onon

- The immune response is a critical factor in the acquisition, progression and clearance of genital warts and cervical neoplasia

- Since cervical cancers are viral in origin, generation of antiviral immunity by human papillomavirus (HPV) vaccination could have major benefits

- The development of a prophylactic and/or therapeutic vaccine would represent a substantial clinical advance

- Prophylactic immunity is antibody-mediated, whereas therapeutic immunity against established infection is mediated by cytotoxic T-cells

- Future studies will address difficulties in evaluating vaccine efficacy

Introduction: Limitations of current treatments and the need for additional therapy

Worldwide, cervical cancer represents a major disease burden, which falls mostly on countries least able to deal with the problem. In developed nations, huge resources are spent on screening women and management of those identified by abnormal smears. Although effective treatment for early cancers exists, the mortality rate for advanced cervical cancer exceeds 50%, and there is a need for improved adjuvant therapy. The situation in developing countries is even more serious; national screening programmes do not exist, women frequently present with advanced disease, and treatment facilities are limited. Most treatments for anogenital warts prevent lesion proliferation, or destroy or excise lesions without specifically targeting the underlying human papillomavirus (HPV) infection. Hence, the potential for recurrence is high, and specific antiviral treatment or prophylaxis would be especially beneficial. Cervical intraepithelial neoplasia (CIN) is now treated effectively and easily by local excision or destruction; however, there is still a degree of morbidity associated with treatment procedures, and the management of recurrent disease is more complex.

These considerations illustrate the potentially enormous health gain which would result from a prophylactic vaccine that could reduce the incidence of cervical cancer by preventing HPV infection, or from a therapeutic vaccine for active treatment.

Immune surveillance in cervical neoplasia

The role of the immune response in limiting cervical cancer development is unproven, but is supported indirectly by the higher incidence of HPV infection, CIN and disease recurrence after treatment in immunocompromised patients. HPV infection and cervical neoplasia are associated with impaired cell-mediated immunity, not disorders of humoral immunity, which implies that cellular immune effectors are more important than antibodies in these diseases.

Further evidence of immunity against HPV disease derives from established and experimental treatments for HPV lesions that appear to work by modifying local immune responses (Table 1). Treatment of genital warts using interferons alpha, beta and gamma in clinical trials produces variable results, with success rates of 15% or less to 81%. The intralesional route is more successful than topical or subcutaneous administration. However, therapy is restricted by cost, the pain that occurs on injection, systemic side-effects and variable efficacy. Interferon can be used in combination with ablative therapy and cytotoxics, and is particularly beneficial after laser surgery.

Table 1 Immune response modifiers can treat HPV lesions

Product	Description	Mechanism
Interferons	Endogenous cytokines acting as the body's first line of defence against major viral diseases	Induction of host-cell antiviral proteins, and immunoregulatory changes
Imiquimod cream (5%)	Topical immune-response modifier for the treatment of external genital warts;[1] under development for CIN[2]	Induction of local interferon secretion, stimulation of T-cell immunity and indirect reduction in HPV load
Cidofovir	Topical antiviral gel	Active metabolite preferentially inhibits viral DNA polymerases
Photodynamic therapy	Topical photosensitizers are under assessment for management of lower genital tract neoplasia[3]	Acts via cellular immune effectors

HPV targets in cervical neoplasia

HPV infection is limited to the epithelium; the viral lifecycle depends on infection of basal cells that normally differentiate into mature squamous cells as they progress towards the epithelial surface. HPV viral particles consist of the viral DNA genome surrounded by the protein capsid, which is composed of HPV L1 and L2 proteins. Thus, it is possible that antibodies against L1 and L2 could be virus-neutralizing, and prevent or attenuate infection.

Once HPV infects, early viral proteins are expressed within lower epithelial layers and viral replication occurs. As infected cells reach the surface, the L1 and L2 proteins are produced and allow shedding of mature virions with exfoliated cells. Cervical HPV infection is usually benign, but its manifestations range from 'warty' epithelium with koilocytosis, to overt malignancy. During infection, HPV DNA is generally found in the cytoplasm. However, the majority of cervical tumours show integration of high-risk (HR) HPV DNA into the host genome, with loss of virion production (L1 and L2 are not expressed). Integration commonly disrupts the HPV virus in the E2 open reading frame; loss of E2 increases expression of E6 and E7, conveying a selective growth advantage to these cells. The net effect of integration is the transformation of infected cells into a malignant phenotype. The constant presence of E6 and E7 in cervical cancers renders them tumour-specific antigens, and raises the possibility that vaccination against E6 and E7 of HR HPV types could produce a therapeutic immune response.

Immune responses to HPV infection and cervical neoplasia

A rational approach to the stimulation of anti-HPV immunity requires knowledge of what immune response, if any, occurs in natural HPV infection. The type of response, and its mechanism, time-course and effects need to be determined. HPV causes no viraemia or systemic manifestations, is not cytolytic and does not activate the inflammatory response. Such chronic infection is more likely to result in immunological tolerance than in T-cell activation. The ability of HPV to persist is consistent with the concept of the virus having low immunogenicity. However, there is almost certainly a role for the immune system in limiting and eradicating HPV infection, and it is this immunity which vaccination seeks to induce or augment.

Humoral immunity

B-lymphocytes mediate humoral immunity through production of immunoglobulins (Ig), leading to destruction of extracellular pathogens. A mature B-cell carries a specific Ig molecule on its surface that recognizes the conformation of a particular antigen (Figure 1). Binding of a receptor Ig molecule to an HPV antigen activates the B-cell, stimulating rapid proliferation, and creates a clone of plasma cells that secrete antibody to the viral antigen. Neutralizing antibodies bind to sites that inactivate the virus.

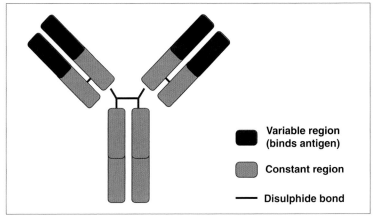

Figure 1 Schematic structure of the immunoglobulin molecule

HPV antibodies may be functionally significant, and possibly markers for monitoring disease progression. However, assays cannot yet distinguish between eradicated and ongoing HPV infection. Several studies have reported an association between HPV 16 antibodies and cervical cancer, with significantly higher seropositivity in patients, compared with controls.[4,5] Seropositivity to HPV 16 E7 may be positively correlated with disease stage and associated with a worse prognosis. The development of HPV antibodies in association with disease progression implies that antibodies are secondary to prolonged antigen exposure and increasing viral load, rather than a mechanism for tumour clearance. This is consistent with the concept that cellular, not humoral, immunity has the critical role of destroying virally infected cells. However, there remains the possibility that antibodies against HPV capsid proteins could neutralize viral particles, preventing or controlling infection. Whilst there are several studies that have associated HPV 16 capsid antibodies with cervical infection by HPV 16, the available data continue to support the view that this is a consequence of persistent exposure to the antigen. There are no longitudinal studies of seropositivity in HPV-negative women, to establish whether capsid antibodies reduce re-infection.

Cellular immunity

Once virus particles have entered host cells, infection is dealt with by cell-mediated immunity, not by antibody. Cytotoxic T-lymphocytes (CTLs) recognize foreign peptide antigens presented on the infected target cell surface by molecules of the major histocompatibility complex (MHC) (also known as human leucocyte antigens, or HLAs). Class I MHC molecules possess an alpha chain with a groove for binding a great variety of peptide antigens (Figure 2), such as those produced by an HPV-infected cell. After peptide binding, the MHC-peptide complex is presented at the cell surface, where, in the presence of co-stimulatory molecules, binding to a CTL may induce an immune response. Individuals with different MHC profiles may vary considerably in their cellular immune responses to the same antigen. This variability is a factor in explaining genetic predisposition to infectious disease, and has implications for the design of therapeutic vaccines.

Multiple animal models of HPV infection have implicated the cellular response in lesion regression. In addition, infiltrating T-cells are seen in regressing warts caused by low-risk (LR) HPVs. Cervical cancers show tumour-infiltrating lymphocytes that are predominantly CTLs. Even high-grade CIN lesions may 'spontaneously' regress in what is, presumably, an immunologically mediated manner. Specific CTLs against HR HPV oncoproteins have been identified in the peripheral blood of patients with cervical cancer and CIN, and also in healthy subjects testing positive for HPV 16.[6] Specific CTLs also infiltrate cervical tumours and are retained in higher numbers at the disease site than in peripheral blood.

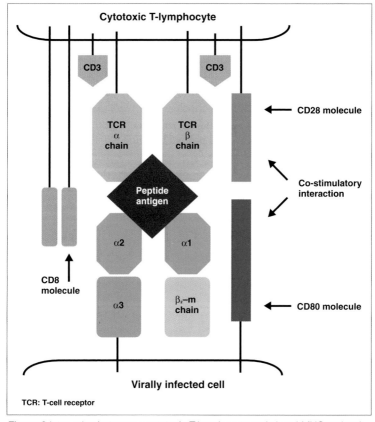

Figure 2 Interaction between a cytotoxic T-lymphocyte and class I MHC molecule

Specific T-cell responses are technically difficult to measure, and although no clear picture of natural HPV immunity has emerged, patients with cervical neoplasia have demonstrated proliferative T-helper (T_H) cell responses to several HPV 16 proteins.[7] There is no definite relationship between immune responsiveness and disease clearance, nor has it been established whether proliferation to HPV 16 E7 is associated with persistent infection, or clearance of HPV and CIN regression. Nevertheless, T_H1 proliferation may generate specific CTLs that could eliminate HPV lesions.

Strategies for vaccine development

Approaches to vaccine development depend on whether a prophylactic or therapeutic response is sought (Table 2). Immunoprophylaxis is a possible approach for genital warts and low-grade neoplasia. Prophylaxis may occur via virus-neutralizing antibodies to prevent infection; specific serum IgG to confer protection by exudation onto mucosal surfaces and inactivation of the pathogen; and secretory IgA molecules to protect the mucosa. For HPV, effective prophylactic vaccination would generate antibodies in genital tract epithelium directed against the L1 and L2 capsid proteins that have a role in viral entry. However, while prophylaxis may be effective, warts and low-grade lesions have little malignant potential and are readily treated by established local methods. Currently, immunotherapy has little relevance in such cases.

Table 2 Vaccination strategies

	Prophylaxis		Therapy
	Genital warts	Low-grade lesions	High-grade lesions
Genotypes	Low risk	Low or high risk	High risk
Viral antigens	L1 L2	L1 L2	E6 E7
Response	Humoral (antibody)	Humoral (antibody)	Cellular (CTLs)

CTLs: Cytotoxic T-lymphocytes

Immunotherapy of malignancy is a more challenging target. Once cervical keratinocytes have undergone transformation, they no longer express HPV late genes and would not bind antibodies directed against capsid proteins. Since continued expression of E6 and E7 is necessary to maintain cells in a transformed state, it is possible that the generation of specific CTLs against HR HPV E6 and/or E7 peptides would lead to the destruction of these infected tumour cells. These concepts support the rationale for continued research into HPV vaccines.

Potential HPV vaccines

Table 3 Candidate HPV vaccines

Type	Characteristic	Response	Prophylaxis	Therapy
Virus-like particles (VLPs)	L1 expressed in culture spontaneously forms virions	Humoral	L1 VLP effective in animal models	Possible (e.g. chimeric E7-L1 VLP)
Recombinant viral vectors	Live attenuated vaccine virus, containing gene-encoding antigen e.g. E6 and E7	Humoral + cellular	Possible	E6 and E7 active in rat model
Recombinant bacterial vectors	e.g. live attenuated *L. monocytogenes* expressing E1	Humoral + cellular	Active in rabbit studies	Possible
Viral DNA	Gene-encoding antigen	Humoral + cellular	Possible	Possible
Proteins	Denatured protein	Humoral + cellular	Possible	Possible chimeric L2E6E7 fusion protein active in mouse model[8]
Peptides	Able to bind to HLA molecules[9]	Cellular	Not known	Possible
Denditric cells (DCs)	DCs loaded with tumour antigens and re-injected[10]	Humoral + cellular	Not known	Possible

CTLs: Cytotoxic T-lymphocytes; HLAs: Human leucocyte antigens

Although the *in vitro* culture of HPV is extremely difficult, because replication is so closely linked to target-cell differentiation, there are several alternative forms in which HPV antigens could be presented by vaccination. The key features of candidate HPV vaccines are shown in Table 3. Of these possible vehicles, recombinant viral vectors have the advantage of inducing antibody responses and stimulating specific CTLs (Figure 3).

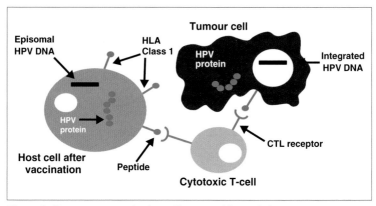

Figure 3 Response to vaccination with a recombinant viral vector

A vaccinia recombinant (TA-HPV) has been used in the first reported study of HPV vaccination in humans.[11] It included HPV 16 and 18 E6 and E7 with modifications to minimize oncogenicity. The ability of vaccinia to replicate in human cells contributes to its immunogenicity and efficiency as a viral vector. However, anti-vector immunity limits the effectiveness of booster vaccinations. The infectivity of vaccinia also increases its adverse-event profile. Therefore, there is a place for vectors which can infect human cells and express their genes, but which are replication-deficient, such as recombinant avian poxviruses.

DNA vaccines are generally less potent than recombinants, presumably because there is no replicative amplification and less inflammation than occurs with attenuated infection. However, their advantages include easy production, stability, induction of both humoral and cellular responses, lack of pathogenicity and potential multivalency of a single vaccine. HPV 16 E6, E7 and L1 plasmid DNA have been used to generate both cell-mediated and antibody responses, with tumour rejection or control.

Clinical trials

Results reported from clinical trials of HPV vaccines in humans are summarized in Table 4. No serious adverse events attributable to virus were seen in any study, and the trials have demonstrated antigenicity. In particular, the study of Koutsky *et al.*, in which 2392 women were randomized to receive three doses of vaccine or placebo, showed a reduced incidence of persistent HPV 16 infection (0 vs 3.8 per 100 women-years at risk) and no cases of HPV 16-related CIN (vs 9 cases in the placebo group).[12] To date, all published trials of HPV vaccines have been Phase I/II studies, in which safety and immunogenicity have been the main concerns. These preliminary results have demonstrated immunogenicity and safety, and further studies are ongoing.[13] Clinical outcomes, however, will be more difficult to measure, since trial endpoints are especially complicated to define.

Table 4 Clinical trials demonstrate antigenicity

Type	Antigen	Disease (n)	Response (n)
Fusion protein[14]	HPV 16 L2 E7 E6	Healthy volunteers (40)	Antibody; T_H response (8)
Virus-like particles[15]	HPV 16 L1	Healthy volunteers (43)	CTL and T_H responses
Dendritic cells[10]	HPV 16 or 18 E7	Cervical cancer (15)	Antibody (3); T_H responses (4)
Recombinant vaccinia virus[16]	HPV 16 & 18; E6 & E7	Vulval intraepithelial neoplasia (VIN) (18)	Antibody (2); T_H responses
Peptide[17]	HPV 16 L2	Healthy volunteers (10)	Antibody (4)
Recombinant vaccinia virus[18]	HPV 16 & 18; E6 & E7	VIN and vaginal IN (VAIN) (12)	T_H responses (6)
Recombinant vaccinia virus[19]	HPV 16 E2	Cervical IN (CIN) (36)	Antibody; CTL
Fusion protein[20]	HPV 16 E7	CIN (7)	Antibody (7); CTL (5); T_H responses (2)
Virus-like particles[21]	HPV 11 or 16 L1	Healthy volunteers	Antibody
Virus-like particles[22]	HPV 18 L1	Healthy volunteers	Antibody

CTL: Cytotoxic T-lymphocyte

Choice of vaccine

Early vaccine studies have focused on HPV 16 antigens, due to the prevalence of HPV 16 in cancer, and lack of diversity across types.[23] Vaccination against LR HPV types would also be beneficial, so further studies are indicated. However, our understanding of HPV population dynamics is far from complete, and it cannot be assumed that vaccination to eliminate infection by certain HPV types will not alter infection rates and/or pathogenicity of other types.[24]

Choice of population

In Phase I safety studies, the trial populations often comprise women with pre-existing infection. However, if a therapeutic vaccine became widely available, it would need to be as effective as existing therapies if it were to be considered for the treatment of CIN. It is possible that vaccination at the time of local treatment might reduce recurrence of CIN; however, since recurrence is already low, very large studies would be required to establish supportive evidence. Vaccination is most unlikely ever to become a primary treatment for cervical cancer, but may prove beneficial as adjuvant therapy. The place of prophylaxis remains equally uncertain and raises the question: should vaccination be offered to sexually active women, to young girls before HPV exposure, or to all individuals for the development of 'herd' immunity? The answer will depend on epidemiological factors, a fuller understanding of the natural history of HPV infection, and the results obtained from large-scale studies such as the NCI Costa Rica study.

Evaluation of vaccine efficacy

The technical problems associated with vaccine evaluation are summarized below. Evaluating HPV vaccines can also be clinically problematic.[25] In order to define trial endpoints, the influence of age and sexual behaviour on HPV acquisition should be taken into account. Other important factors are the latency of HPV infection; its high clearance rate; the long time-course from infection to development of CIN; the frequency with which low-grade cervical lesions regress; and uncertainty about the time taken for CIN to become invasive. All these factors complicate the design of Phase III studies, where clinical endpoints are required.

Problems in detection of HPV antibodies	Problems in evaluating cell-mediated immunity
• Suitable antigenic targets for *in vitro* assay must be synthesized • Procedures are technically difficult and time-consuming • Neutralizing antibodies (active) must be distinguished from binding antibodies (non-active) • Neutralizing antibodies must be quantified for prophylactic vaccine	• HPV-infected cells are required as targets • CTLs are HLA-restricted, so targets must be HLA-compatible • Establishing a subject-specific autologous cell line to provide HLA-matched targets is labour-intensive and unsuited to large-scale trials • Measurement of cytokine production in response to antigen is simpler and sensitive but is rarely used in HPV vaccine trials[21]

There are also many additional factors to consider when developing HPV vaccines for widespread use: safety; cost and timescale of production; stability of the formulation; ease of administration and immunogenicity of single doses. Vaccination formulations or protocols that are acceptable for Phase I trials may not be realistic on a large scale. In addition, any vaccine to be used globally should be stable without refrigeration.

Potential obstacles to effective vaccination

HPV vaccination may fail to achieve effective immunity and, even if an immune response can be induced, the HPV lesion may be able to evade this response.

HPV variants

The multiplicity of HPV types is well known, but within types there may also be variants where up to 2% of the E6, E7 and L1 gene sequences differ from the wild-type. A variant HPV 16 E6 epitope has been identified that may impair CTL recognition of infected cells, and which is associated with fewer antibody responses to HPV 16 L1 virus-like particles than wild type. These findings suggest that there may be mutations other than that of the E6 gene. Any effective vaccine must be active across as many HPV variants as possible.

Immune escape

HPV is purely intraepithelial, with inherently poor immunogenicity, possibly because of the poor expression of co-stimulatory molecules (e.g. CD80), and may not lead to appropriate immune activation in peripheral lymphoid tissues. Even if specific immunity can be generated by vaccination, there are mechanisms by which HPV lesions can evade immunosurveillance, such as effector-cell dysfunction or tumour HLA loss.

Immunity can be impaired by any systemic disease, and may be compromised even in early cervical cancer. Proponents of the immune surveillance theory might argue that progressive tumour development is in itself evidence of functional immunodeficiency; however, the precise causes of immunosuppression have yet to be fully defined.

In many tumours, HLA class I molecules are frequently lost from the cell surface.[26] HLA loss has been reported in the majority of cervical cancers, and also in CIN where it acts as a marker of disease progression.

Since HLA molecules are necessary for viral antigen presentation to T-lymphocytes, their loss has critical implications for immune recognition. Peptide antigens cannot be presented on the tumour-cell surface, so the lesion is not a target for specific CTLs and thus evades cellular immunity. HLA loss may be a selective process that enables cervical neoplasia to progress despite the presence of immune effectors. It may be possible to up-regulate HLA expression and render tumours susceptible to vaccine-induced CTLs, but the variety of mechanisms that cause HLA loss will limit the success of such an approach. Because HLA loss occurs early in the natural history of cervical neoplasia, the development of effective therapeutic HPV vaccination may be precluded. Ultimately, prophylactic vaccination may be the only effective means of inducing beneficial immune responses.

Conclusions

- HPV vaccination can induce lesion regression in animal models

- Preliminary clinical trials of HPV vaccines demonstrate immunogenicity and (short-term) safety

- Measurable CTL and antibody responses can be generated in women with cervical cancer

- The difficulties of inducing a measurable immune response in a consistent, reliable manner should be addressed by the systematic investigation of formulation, route of administration, immunization schedule and host factors

- HPV is exceptionally difficult to vaccinate against because of the multiplicity of types, variants within a type, poor inherent immunogenicity and an association with HLA loss

- It is imperative that clinical trials of HPV vaccines continue; the ultimate question of clinical efficacy remains to be answered

References

1. Edwards L, Ferenczy A, Eron L et al. Self-administered topical 5% imiquimod cream for external anogenital warts. HPV Study Group. Human PapillomaVirus. Arch Dermatol 1998;134:25–30

2. Diaz-Arrastia C, Arany I, Robazetti SC et al. Clinical and molecular responses in high-grade intraepithelial neoplasia treated with topical imiquimod 5%. Clin Cancer Res 2001;7:3031–3

3. Martin-Hirsch P, Kitchener HC, Hampson IN. Photodynamic therapy of lower genital tract neoplasia. Gynecol Oncol 2002;84:187–9

4. Park JS, Park DC, Kim CJ et al. HPV 16-related proteins as the serologic markers in cervical neoplasia. Gynecol Oncol 1998;69:47–55

5. Wang SS, Schiffman M, Shields TS et al. Seroprevalence of human papillomavirus 16, 18, 31 and 45 in a population-based cohort of 10000 women in Costa Rica. Br J Cancer 2003;89:1248–54

6. Konya J, Dillner J. Immunity to oncogenic human papillomaviruses. Adv Cancer Res 2001;82:205–38

7. Stern PL, Brown M, Stacey SN et al. Natural HPV immunity and vaccination strategies. J Clin Virol 2000;19:57–66

8. van der Burg SH, Kwappenberg KM, O'Neill T et al. Pre-clinical safety and efficacy of TA-CIN, a recombinant HPV16 L2E6E7 fusion protein vaccine, in homologous and heterologous prime-boost regimens. Vaccine 2001; 19:3652–60

9. Melief CJ, Kast WM. T-cell immunotherapy of tumors by adoptive transfer of cytotoxic T lymphocytes and by vaccination with minimal essential epitopes. Immunol Rev 1995;145:167–77

10. Ferrara A, Nonn M, Sehr P et al. Dendritic cell-based tumor vaccine for cervical cancer II: results of a clinical pilot study in 15 individual patients. J Cancer Res Clin Oncol 2003;129:521–30

11. Borysiewicz LK, Fiander A, Nimako M et al. A recombinant vaccinia virus encoding human papillomavirus types 16 and 18, E6 and E7 proteins as immunotherapy for cervical cancer. Lancet 1996;347:1523–7

12. Koutsky LA, Ault KA, Wheeler CM et al. A controlled trial of a human papillomavirus type 16 vaccine. N Engl J Med 2002;347:1645–51

13. Adams M, Borysiewicz L, Fiander A et al. Clinical studies of human papilloma vaccines in pre-invasive and invasive cancer. Vaccine 2001;19:2549–56

14. de Jong A, O'Neill T, Khan AY et al. Enhancement of human papillomavirus (HPV) type 16 E6 and E7-specific T cell immunity in healthy volunteers through vaccination with TA-CIN, an HPV16 L2E7E6 fusion protein vaccine. Vaccine 2002;20:3456–64

15. Pinto LA, Edwards J, Castle PE et al. Cellular immune responses to human papillomavirus (HPV) 16 L1 in healthy volunteers immunized with recombinant HPV 16 L1 virus-like particles. J Infect Dis 2003;188:327–38

16. Davidson EJ, Boswell CM, Sehr P et al. Immunological and clinical responses in women with vulval intraepithelial neoplasia vaccinated with a vaccinia virus encoding human papillomavirus 16/18 oncoproteins. Cancer Res 2003;63:6032–41

17. Kawana K, Yasugi T, Kanda T et al. Safety and immunogenicity of a peptide containing the cross-neutralization epitope of HPV16 L2 administered nasally in healthy volunteers. Vaccine 2003;21:4256–60

18. Baldwin PJ, van der Burg SH, Boswell CM et al. Vaccinia-expressed human papillomavirus 16 and 18 E6 and E7 as a therapeutic vaccination for vulval and vaginal intraepithelial neoplasia. Clin Cancer Res 2003;9:5205–13.

19. Corona Gutierrez CM, Tinoco A, Navarro T et al. Therapeutic vaccination with MVA E2 can eliminate precancerous lesions (CIN 1, CIN 2, and CIN 3) associated with infection by oncogenic human papillomavirus. Hum Gene Ther 2004;15:421–31

20. Hallez S, Simon P, Madous F et al. Phase I/II trial of immunogenicity of a human papillomavirus (HPV) type 16 E7 protein-based vaccine in women with oncogenic HPV-positive cervical intraepithelial neoplasia. Cancer Immunol Immunother 2004;53:642–50

21. Fife KH, Wheeler CM, Koutsky LA et al. Dose-ranging studies of the safety and immunogenicity of human papillomavirus type 11 and type 16 virus-like particle candidate vaccines in young healthy women. Vaccine 2004;22:2943–52

22. Ault KA, Giuliano AR, Edwards RP et al. A phase I study to evaluate a human papillomavirus (HPV) type 18 VLP vaccine. Vaccine 2004;22:3004–7

23. Munoz N. Human papillomavirus and cancer: the epidemiological evidence. J Clin Virol 2000;19:1–5

24. Goldie SJ, Grima D, Kohli M et al. A comprehensive natural history model of HPV infection and cancer to estimate the clinical impact of a prophylactic HPV vaccine. Int J Cancer 2003;106:896–904

25. Kang M, Lagakos SW. Evaluating the role of human papillomavirus vaccine in cervical cancer prevention. Stat Methods Med Res 2004;13:139–55

26. Garrido F, Algarra I. MHC antigens and tumor escape from immune surveillance. Adv Cancer Res 2001;83:117–58

5. Molecular markers in cervical dyskaryosis

Niamh Murphy, Martina Ring, Orla Sheils and John O'Leary

- The molecular basis of HPV carcinogenesis is now being unravelled

- Testing for HPV oncogenic activity using marker expression is under investigation

- These markers are:

  - Minichromosome maintenance proteins MCM5 and MCM7
  - The DNA licensing protein, CDC6
  - The tumour suppressor, p16^{INK4A}

Introduction

Cervical screening programmes using Pap smear testing have dramatically improved cervical cancer incidence and reduced deaths, but cervical cancer still remains a global health burden. Despite its success, the single Pap smear test has limited sensitivity and specificity.

Limitations of Pap smear screening

Cytology can give false-positive and false-negative results

- The degree of dyskaryosis in sampled cells may not correspond to histological confirmation of cancer

- Errors in sampling, slide preparation and interpretation are inherent in cytology

- Sampling for atypical glandular cells is exceptionally difficult

- False-positive rates range from 15–50%

- False-negative rates may reach 30%

False-negative and false-positive screening results have serious medical, financial and legal implications. Consequently, more specific methods for testing are required. With the development of molecular marker analysis, the genomic chaos caused by oncogenic HPV infections is now being unravelled, and this knowledge can hopefully be used to improve cervical screening concepts and technologies. This chapter aims to critically assess the present and future role of molecular markers in cervical screening and cancer diagnosis.

The role of HPV in the pathogenesis of cervical cancer

Chapters 1 and 3 describe in detail the role of HPV in the pathogenesis of cervical cancer and how the key HPV oncogenic proteins E6 and E7 interfere with critical cell-cycle pathways.

HPV as a molecular marker of cervical dyskaryosis

High-risk HPV DNA is a marker for current or subsequent development of precursor lesions. Persistent HPV DNA type-specificity is an even stronger predictive factor.[1–3] HPV DNA testing in conjunction with the Pap test is currently being reviewed in the triage of inconclusive or minimally abnormal smears, and as a stand-alone test in primary screening. The HPV DNA test may also have a role in follow-up after ablation for cervical dysplasia, as discussed in Book 2. The persistence of HPV DNA after treatment could be an accurate predictor of residual disease or relapse.

HPV protein, DNA and mRNA testing

Several methods exist for the detection, typing and quantitation of HPV. Commercially available HPV antibodies can be employed for the detection of HPV proteins using techniques such as immuno-histochemistry, western blotting and immunoprecipitation. However, it is difficult to detect the HPV oncoproteins themselves, firstly because of insufficiently sensitive and specific monoclonal antibodies and, secondly, because of the very short half-life and turnover rate of E6 and E7 gene products. Consequently, the standard practical methods for the diagnosis of HPV infection are based on the detection of HPV DNA.

The incorporation of HPV DNA testing into primary screening remains controversial, however. The great majority of HPV infections are transient and clinically non-significant, although they frequently produce temporary cytologic changes. Only 10–20% of HPV infections become persistent and contribute to the development of high-grade precancerous lesions or cervical cancer.[4,5] This is particularly relevant to women in their teens and 20s. It is possible that widespread use of HPV DNA testing will result in the identification of large numbers of women at risk, even though their infections are likely to be transient. Such misclassification would result in over-treatment of lesions, unnecessary expenditure and considerable anxiety for patients.

Testing for HPV oncogenic activity, rather than for the presence of HPV DNA, may therefore be a more relevant clinical indicator of the development of cervical lesions and cervical cancer. The detection of HPV E6/E7 mRNA indicates HPV oncogenic activity and may be used as a clinically predictive marker to identify women at risk of developing high-grade cervical dysplastic lesions and cervical carcinoma.

Host molecular markers of cervical dyskaryosis

HPV infection causes changes in expression of host cervical cell-cycle regulatory proteins. Such differentially expressed host proteins and nucleic acids may have a role as 'biomarkers' of dysplastic cells. Investigation of potential biomarkers may also help to unravel new pathways involved in the HPV-mediated pathogenesis of cervical dyskaryosis. These specific molecular biomarkers will also facilitate the testing of virus-like particle vaccines and other HPV vaccines.[6]

To date, many molecular markers have been evaluated for their role in cervical screening (Table 1). Of these, proliferating cell nuclear antigen (PCNA), the proliferation marker, Ki-67, and hTERT, the small subunit of the cancer-associated enzyme, DNA telomerase,[7] have shown only limited potential.

Conversely, three markers have shown high potential; the DNA replication licensing proteins CDC6 and MCM5[8–11] and the cyclin-dependent kinase inhibitor p16^{INK4A}.[12,13]

Table 1 Molecular markers used in cervical cancer screening

	Type	Limitation
PCNA	Proliferation marker	Multiple factors affect staining intensity
Ki-67	Proliferation marker	Multiple factors affect expression levels
hTERT	Telomerase small subunit	False-positive and false-negative results

Minichromosome maintenance proteins

DNA replication occurs only once in a single normal cell cycle, due to a mechanism known as 'licensing' of DNA replication.[14] This process requires the assembly of a protein complex which includes the cell division cycle protein 6 (CDC6) and the minichromosome maintenance (MCM) proteins.[15,16] Disassembly of this complex prevents repetitive replication during the same cell cycle.[17]

Changes in the expression pattern of DNA 'licensing' proteins are frequently observed in dysplastic cells. In normal cells, MCM5 and CDC6 are present only during the cell cycle and are lost from the cell during quiescence and differentiation. However, marked over-expression of MCM proteins and CDC6 are observed in dysplastic cells. MCM5 and CDC6 have, therefore, been proposed as specific biomarkers of proliferating cells.

MCM proteins as markers of cervical dysplasia

In normal cervical epithelium, MCM protein staining is limited to the basal proliferating layer and is absent in differentiated and quiescent cells.[9,11] In cervical glandular and squamous dysplasia, however, MCM expression is dramatically increased, suggesting its potential as a biomarker of cervical dysplasia.[18–23] MCM5 has been the focus of much of this research, but MCM7 is also a highly informative marker of cervical cancer.[9,24] The number of nuclei positive for MCM5 at the surface of dysplastic epithelium correlates with the severity of dysplasia.[9,11]

Figure 1 illustrates MCM5 immunohistochemical staining in cervical squamous and glandular lesions, invasive squamous cell carcinoma and adenocarcinoma of the cervix. MCM5 also stains exfoliated dysplastic cells on liquid-based cytology slides and has potential as a marker of exfoliated dysplastic cells. A striking increase in MCM5 protein expression is observed in cells showing histological HPV features.

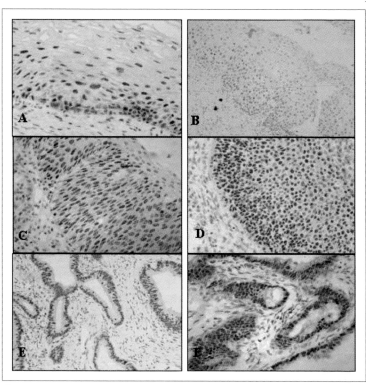

Figure 1 Immunohistochemical staining for MCM5 in (A) CIN 1; (B) CIN 1-2; (C) CIN 3; (D) invasive squamous cell carcinoma of the cervix; (E) cervical glandular intraepithelial neoplasia (cGIN); and (F) adenocarcinoma of the cervix

MCM5 and HPV oncoprotein expression

- MCM5 overexpression may be due to the release of Rb inhibition on transcription factor E2F due to binding of HPV E7 oncoproteins

- E2F may bind to the MCM5 promoter to increase transcription of MCM5

- Our results show that MCM5 mRNA expression (by real-time PCR) increases significantly with increasing severity of dysplasia

CDC6 as a marker of cervical dyskaryosis

CDC6 protein expression is also present in proliferating cells, but is absent in differentiated or quiescent cells. In normal cervical epithelium, CDC6 staining is absent or limited to the basal proliferative layer. However, CDC6 protein expression is dramatically up-regulated in squamous and glandular cervical carcinomas.

CDC6 was first identified in 1998 as a marker of cervical dysplastic cells in cervical biopsies and in smears using polyclonal antibodies.[9] In subsequent studies (Bonds *et al.*, 2002 and our own group), it was observed that CDC6 stains high-grade cervical lesions, although the proportion of positively stained lesional cells was lower than that previously reported.[8] In lower-grade lesions, CDC6 protein expression is weak or absent. CDC6 was preferentially expressed in areas exhibiting histological HPV changes.

Interestingly, the expression pattern of CDC6 closely mirrors that of the high-risk HPV E6 oncoprotein, which is mainly expressed in higher-grade lesions and invasive carcinomas. In this context, CDC6 overexpression appears to be a relatively late event in the 'dysplastic progression model'.

CDC6 and HPV oncoprotein expression

- Inactivation of Rb by HPV E7
  - Releases inhibition of E2F
  - May transcriptionally up-regulate CDC6

- Our results show that CDC6 mRNA expression (by real-time PCR) is significantly increased in high-grade dysplastic cells

- Overexpression of CDC6 promotes re-replication, genomic instability and DNA damage in human cancer cells with inactive p53, but not in cells with functional p53

- High-risk HPV E6 oncoprotein targets p53 for proteolytic degradation, allowing re-replication to occur in the presence of CDC6 overexpression

$p16^{INK4A}$

The CDKN2A gene located on chromosome 9p21 encodes the tumour suppressor protein, $p16^{INK4A}$. This 16 kDa protein inhibits cyclin-dependent kinases 4 and 6 (Figure 2).

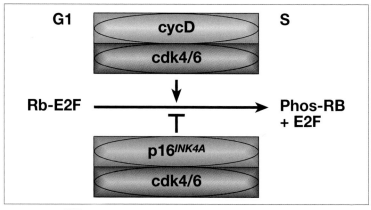

Figure 2 $p16^{INK4A}$ and the retinoblastoma pathway; cell-cycle progression is inhibited by $p16^{INK4A}$

Unsurprisingly, loss of p16^{INK4A} function represents a common pathway to tumourigenesis. p16^{INK4A} can be inactivated by a variety of genetic alterations including mutation, altered splicing, homozygous deletion[25] and promoter hypermethylation.[26] However, overexpression of p16^{INK4A} protein in tumours has also been described.

p16^{INK4A} as a marker of cervical dyskaryosis

The expression pattern of p16^{INK4A} in dysplastic squamous and glandular cervical cells in tissue sections and in cervical smears has been extensively investigated.[12,27–32] In all normal cervical tissues examined, no p16^{INK4A} staining is evident. In addition, all normal regions adjacent to cervical intraepithelial neoplasia (CIN) lesions do not show any detectable p16^{INK4A} expression. In cervical biopsy sections, p16^{INK4A} identified dysplastic squamous and glandular lesions with a sensitivity rate of 99.9% and a specificity rate of 100%.[30] Figure 3 illustrates p16^{INK4A} immunostaining in squamous and glandular lesions and in invasive squamous cell carcinoma and adenocarcinoma of the cervix. Figure 4 illustrates p16^{INK4A} staining in exfoliated dysplastic cells.

---

p16^{INK4A} and HPV oncoprotein expression

- Inactivation of Rb by HPV E7 protein may up-regulate p16^{INK4A}

- p16^{INK4A} may be directly induced by the transcription factor E2F released from pRb after binding of HPV E7

- A significant increase in p16^{INK4A} protein expression is seen in:
  - HPV-associated penile carcinomas
  - HPV-associated oral cancers

- An HPV-independent pathway for p16^{INK4A} up-regulation may also exist

---

It is now widely accepted that p16^{INK4A} is a sensitive and specific marker of squamous and glandular dysplastic cells of the cervix and is a valuable adjunctive test in cervical cancer screening. A study

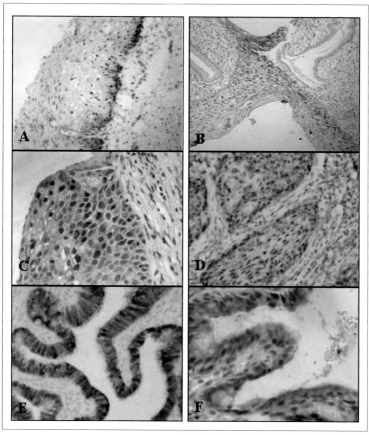

Figure 3 Immunohistochemical staining for p16^{INK4A} in (A) CIN 1; (B) CIN 2; (C) CIN 3; (D) invasive squamous cell carcinoma; (E) cGIN; and (F) adenocarcinoma of the cervix

published by Klaes *et al.*, 2002, in which five experienced pathologists participated, clearly demonstrated that the use of p16^{INK4A} immunostaining allows the precise identification of CIN and cervical cancer lesions in cervical biopsy specimens and can significantly reduce false-negative and false-positive results in cervical cancer screening.[33]

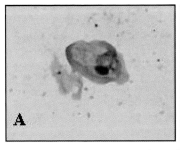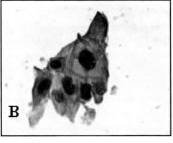

Figure 4 Immunocytochemical staining of exfoliated dyplastic cells in ThinPrep® slides using p16^{INK4A} specific antibody; p16^{INK4A} expression in (A) a mild dyskaryotic cell; and (B) a mild to moderately dyskaryotic cell cluster

For the accurate use of p16^{INK4A} in the detection of adenocarcinoma and its precursor lesions, knowledge of p16^{INK4A} staining patterns is essential.

Differential characteristics of tubo-endometroid metaplasia (TEM)

- A benign histological lesion where endometrial or fallopian tube-type cells are present in the endocervical glands, due to metaplasia

- Can give rise to diagnostic difficulty when found at the transformation zone

- TEM may be histologically misinterpreted as cervical glandular intraepithelial neoplasia (cGIN) or adenocarcinoma *in situ* (AIS)

    - Occasional p16^{INK4A} nuclear positivity and definite cytoplasmic staining

    - Intercalating tubal/peg cells are negative for p16^{INK4A} expression

    - These TEM p16^{INK4A} staining patterns are distinct from the intense nuclear and cytoplasmic staining observed in cGIN p16^{INK4A} also stains endosalpingiosis and fallopian tube epithelium, thus creating two other potential diagnostic pitfalls. Cameron *et al.*, 2002, have suggested using a panel of antibodies composed of p16^{INK4A}, MIB1 and bcl2 to discriminate problematic endocervical glandular lesions.[34] Such a panel would be able to distinguish cGIN from TEM, endometriosis or microglandular hyperplasia.

Conclusions

- Oncogenic HPV infection causes changes in expression of host cell-cycle regulatory proteins

- MCM5, CDC6 and $p16^{INK4A}$ expression can be used as markers of dysplasia

- Our increasing knowledge of the pathogenesis of cervical cancer combined with advances in microarray technologies heralds the emergence of a 'molecular age' in cervical cancer prevention

- This new era promises the identification and characterization of novel biomarkers of cervical dysplasia

- The use of biomarkers in conjunction with conventional screening and HPV testing will ultimately result in a reduction in patient anxiety, and in the overall cost of cervical cancer screening

- These biomarkers will also help to further define the pathogenesis of HPV infection and dysplastic progression

References

1. Bosch FX, de Sanjose S. Human papillomavirus and cervical cancer – burden and assessment of causality. *J Natl Cancer Inst Monogr* 2003:3–13

2. Munoz N, Bosch FX, de Sanjose S *et al*. Epidemiologic classification of human papillomavirus types associated with cervical cancer. *N Engl J Med* 2003;348:518–27

3. Schiffman M, Herrero R, Hildesheim A *et al*. HPV DNA testing in cervical cancer screening: results from women in a high-risk province of Costa Rica. *JAMA* 2000;283:87–93

4. Remmink AJ, Walboomers JM, Helmerhorst TJ *et al*. The presence of persistent high-risk HPV genotypes in dysplastic cervical lesions is associated with progressive disease: natural history up to 36 months. *Int J Cancer* 1995;61:306–11

5. Ho GY, Burk RD, Klein S *et al*. Persistent genital human papillomavirus infection as a risk factor for persistent cervical dysplasia. *J Natl Cancer Inst* 1995;87:1365–71

6. Fausch SC, Da Silva DM, Eiben GL *et al*. HPV protein/peptide vaccines: from animal models to clinical trials. *Front Bioscience* 2003;8:81–91

7. Jarboe EA, Liaw KL, Thompson LC *et al*. Analysis of telomerase as a diagnostic biomarker of cervical dysplasia and carcinoma. *Oncogene* 2002;21:664–73

8. Bonds L, Baker P, Gup C, Shroyer KR. Immunohistochemical localization of cdc6 in squamous and glandular neoplasia of the uterine cervix. *Arch Pathol Lab Med* 2002;126:1164–8

9. Williams GH, Romanowski P, Morris L *et al*. Improved cervical smear assessment using antibodies against proteins that regulate DNA replication. *Proc Natl Acad Sci U S A* 1998;95:14932–7

10. Fujita M, Yamada C, Goto H *et al*. Cell cycle regulation of human CDC6 protein. Intracellular localization, interaction with the human mcm complex, and CDC2 kinase-mediated hyperphosphorylation. *J Biol Chem* 1999; 274:25927–32

11. Freeman A, Morris LS, Mills AD *et al*. Minichromosome maintenance proteins as biological markers of dysplasia and malignancy. *Clin Cancer Res* 1999;5:2121–32

12. Klaes R, Friedrich T, Spitkovsky D *et al*. Overexpression of p16(INK4A) as a specific marker for dysplastic and neoplastic epithelial cells of the cervix uteri. *Int J Cancer* 2001;92:276–84

13. Murphy NB, Pelle R. The use of arbitrary primers and the RADES method for the rapid identification of developmentally regulated genes in trypanosomes. *Gene* 1994;141:53–61

14. Takisawa H, Mimura S, Kubota Y. Eukaryotic DNA replication: from pre-replication complex to initiation complex. *Curr Opin Cell Biol* 2000;12:690–6

15. Shin JH, Grabowski B, Kasiviswanathan R *et al*. Regulation of minichromosome maintenance helicase activity by Cdc6. *J Biol Chem* 2003;278:38059–67

16. Cook JG, Park CH, Burke TW *et al*. Analysis of Cdc6 function in the assembly of mammalian prereplication complexes. *Proc Natl Acad Sci U S A* 2002;99:1347–52

17. Lei M, Tye BK. Initiating DNA synthesis: from recruiting to activating the MCM complex. *J Cell Sci* 2001;114:1447–54

18. Stoeber K, Swinn R, Prevost AT *et al*. Diagnosis of genito-urinary tract cancer by detection of minichromosome maintenance 5 protein in urine sediments. *J Natl Cancer Inst* 2002;94:1071–9

19. Going JJ, Keith WN, Neilson L *et al*. Aberrant expression of minichromosome maintenance proteins 2 and 5, and Ki-67 in dysplastic squamous oesophageal epithelium and Barrett's mucosa. *Gut* 2002;50:373–7

20. Alison MR, Hunt T, Forbes SJ. Minichromosome maintenance (MCM) proteins may be pre-cancer markers. *Gut* 2002;50:290–1

21. Davies RJ, Freeman A, Morris LS *et al*. Analysis of minichromosome maintenance proteins as a novel method for detection of colorectal cancer in stool. *Lancet* 2002;359:1917–9

22. Ohta S, Koide M, Tokuyama T *et al*. Cdc6 expression as a marker of proliferative activity in brain tumors. *Oncol Rep* 2001;8:1063–6

23. Davidson EJ, Morris LS, Scott IS *et al*. Minichromosome maintenance (Mcm) proteins, cyclin B1 and D1, phosphohistone H3 and in situ DNA replication for functional analysis of vulval intraepithelial neoplasia. *Br J Cancer* 2003;88:257–62

24. Brake T, Connor JP, Petereit DG, Lambert PF. Comparative analysis of cervical cancer in women and in a human papillomavirus-transgenic mouse model: identification of minichromosome maintenance protein 7 as an informative biomarker for human cervical cancer. *Cancer Res* 2003;63:8173–80

25. Kamb A, Gruis NA, Weaver-Feldhaus J *et al*. A cell cycle regulator potentially involved in genesis of many tumor types. *Science* 1994;264:436–40

26. Merlo A, Herman JG, Mao L et al. 5' CpG island methylation is associated with transcriptional silencing of the tumour suppressor p16/CDKN2/MTS1 in human cancers. Nat Med 1995;1:686–92

27. Bibbo M, Klump WJ, DeCecco J, Kovatich AJ. Procedure for immunocytochemical detection of P16^{INK4A} antigen in thin-layer, liquid-based specimens. Acta Cytologica 2002;46:25–9

28. Negri G, Egarter-Vigl E, Kasal A et al. p16^{INK4A} is a useful marker for the diagnosis of adenocarcinoma of the cervix uteri and its precursors: an immunohistochemical study with immunocytochemical correlations. Am J Surg Pathol 2003;27:187–93

29. Pientong C, Ekalaksananan T, Swadpanich U et al. Immunocytochemical detection of p16^{INK4A} protein in scraped cervical cells. Acta Cytologica 2003;47:616–23

30. Murphy N, Ring M, Killalea AG et al. p16^{INK4A} as a marker for cervical dyskaryosis: CIN and cGIN in cervical biopsies and ThinPrep smears. J Clin Pathol 2003;56:56–63

31. Saqi A, Pasha TL, McGrath CM et al. Overexpression of p16^{INK4A} in liquid-based specimens (SurePath) as marker of cervical dysplasia and neoplasia. Diagn Cytopathol 2002;27:365–70

32. Sano T, Oyama T, Kashiwabara K et al. Immunohistochemical over-expression of p16 protein associated with intact retinoblastoma protein expression in cervical cancer and cervical intraepithelial neoplasia. Pathol Int 1998;48:580–5

33. Klaes R, Benner A, Friedrich T et al. p16^{INK4A} immunohistochemistry improves interobserver agreement in the diagnosis of cervical intraepithelial neoplasia. Am J Surg Pathol 2002;26:1389–99

34. Cameron RI, Maxwell P, Jenkins D, McCluggage WG. Immunohistochemical staining with MIB1, bcl2 and p16 assists in the distinction of cervical glandular intraepithelial neoplasia from tubo-endometrial metaplasia, endometriosis and microglandular hyperplasia. Histopathology 2002;41:313–21

Index